Infection Control for Lodging and Food Service Establishments

Infection Control for Lodging and Food Service Establishments

John Jefferson Dykstra
The J.D. Group, Inc.
Infection Control Training Center

WILEY

John Wiley & Sons, Inc.
New York • Chichester • Brisbane • Toronto • Singapore

Copyright © 1990 by John Wiley & Sons, Inc.
All rights reserved. Published simultaneously in Canada.
Reproduction or translation of any part of this work beyond that permitted by section 107 or 108 of the 1976 United States Copyright Act without the permission of the copyright owner is unlawful. Requests for permission or further information should be addressed to the Permission Department, John Wiley & Sons, Inc.

Library of Congress Cataloging-in-Publication Data

Dykstra, John Jefferson
   Infection control for lodging and food service establishments / John Jefferson Dykstra

ISBN 0-471-62317-2

Printed in the United States of America
90 91 10 9 8 7 6 5 4 3 2 1

Contents

363.7296
D996i

Introduction   1

Chapter 1: The Need for Infection Control   9
    World Travel   9
    The Sex and Drug Revolutions   10
    The Aging of America   10
    THE NEED FOR INFECTION CONTROL   11
    THE MARKETING ADVANTAGE   14
    SUMMARY   15
    REVIEW EXERCISES   16

Chapter 2: Fundamentals, Glossary, and
            Definitions   17
    UNDERSTANDING THE BASICS:
        A GLOSSARY   18
    MICROBIAL LIFE   19
    MODES AND ROUTES OF
        TRANSMISSION   25
        Cross-contamination   25
    SUMMARY   30
    REVIEW EXERCISES   30

Chapter 3: Relevant Diseases   33
    HEPATITIS   35
    LEGIONNELLOSIS (LEGIONNAIRES'
        DISEASE)   36
    HERPES SIMPLEX I AND II   38
    AIDS   39

SALMONELLA   43
TUBERCULOSIS   44
THE IMPORTANCE OF INFECTION CONTROL
    TO EMPLOYERS AND EMPLOYEES   44
SUMMARY   46
REVIEW EXERCISES   46

Chapter 4: The Employee and Infection Control   49
CLOTHING   51
HAND WASHING   51
SCREENING FOR RISK   53
SUMMARY   61
REVIEW EXERCISES   62

Chapter 5: Environmental Surface Disinfectants   63
DISINFECTANTS   65
PRECLEANING   66
CHOOSING A PRODUCT   67
LAWS AND REGULATIONS CONCERNING
    DISINFECTANTS   68
    Definitions   69
    Federal Agencies   69
    Misleading Labels and Unsupported
        Claims   71
CAVEAT EMPTOR—BUYER, BEWARE!   73
DISINFECTANT REVIEW   76
    Disinfection Product Applications   77
INFECTION-CONTROL PRODUCT UPDATE:
    TECHNOLOGY BREAKTHROUGH   77
QUATERNARY AMMONIUM COMPOUNDS:
    "SUPER QUATS"   81
SUMMARY   82
REVIEW EXERCISES   83

Chapter 6: Guest Room Disinfection   85
IMPROVING GUEST ROOM
    DISINFECTION   90
    A Scenario   92
    Beyond "Clean"   92
    Avoiding Risk   95

Introducing Disinfectant Products   96
AVOIDING LIABILITY AND ADVERSE
     PUBLICITY   97
     High Stakes, Simple Precautions   98
SUMMARY   101
REVIEW EXERCISES   101

Chapter 7: Food and Beverage Areas   103
SCENARIO—THE NASTY WAITRESS   105
SANITATION-RELATED TASKS   105
SANITATION TRAINING FOR COOKS AND
     CHEFS   106
TRAY CLEANING   109
BAR/LOUNGE/FOOD AREAS   109
     Situation 1   109
     Situation 2   110
     Scenario   110
CIRCULATION AND DISINFECTION OF
     UTENSILS AND GLASSWARE   112
     Situation   112
     Solution   112
THE THREE-SINK THEORY   113
     The Wash Tank, Rinse Tank, and Sanitize
     Tank   113
INFECTION CONTROL FOR FOOD SERVICE
     OPERATIONS   115
     Example 1   115
     Example 2   116
SUMMARY   125
REVIEW EXERCISES   126

Chapter 8: Marketing Infection Control   129
REACHING THE CUSTOMER   131
MARKETING IDEAS: LODGING
     ESTABLISHMENTS   131
     Group 1   131
     Group 2   131
     Group 3   132
MARKETING IDEAS: RESTAURANTS   133

SUMMARY   135
REVIEW EXERCISES   135

Chapter 9: OSHA Employee Compliance
            Training   137
OSHA INSPECTIONS   139
REVIEW QUESTIONS   157

Review Self-test   159

References   165

Bibliography   167

Answers to Review Questions   169

Index   173

Acknowledgment

I wish to thank all those people I had an opportunity to learn from and work with to make this concept a reality.

Preface

This book is designed to alert lodging and food service personnel to the potential impact of infectious diseases, the risk of cross-contamination, and the need for infection-control programs throughout the hospitality industry.

The effects of Legionnaires' disease and Hepatitis A within the hospitality industry are well documented. The possible risks posed by other diseases, including AIDS, are less well known. An infection-control program is not only a wise policy from the standpoint of avoiding health risks, but can also be an effective marketing strategy for those individual properties or corporations that seize the initiative.

The primary objectives of this book are:

1. To make hospitality personnel and management aware of cross-infection risk factors that currently exist and to emphasize that these factors will increase as more and more people present themselves in lodging and food service facilities.

2. To provide a marketing tool for the ability to allay public fears regarding risk of disease transmission in lodging and food service establishments.

3. To describe a simple, easy-to-implement, cost-effective program of infection control that can be utilized by housekeeping and food service personnel.

4. To provide generic product information which will assist purchasing personnel in making product evaluations.

5. To offer a learning aid that can be used by newly hired housekeeping and food service personnel, as well as by management.

The information presented in this book is based on that offered in educational programs offered by the J.D. Group as a means of reducing the risk of contagious disease to the public and hospitality industry employees.

Introduction

The food service industry has experienced a phenomenal number of disease-related outbreaks. It is nationally recognized that only five to ten percent of food-related illnesses are reported to local environmental agencies and that the real number of illnesses is at least 25 times that reported. The Food and Drug Administration (FDA) feels greater efforts should be made to determine the incidences of all diarrheal and food-borne diarrheal disease.

In the hospitality industry, the process of eliminating disease-causing organisms is often taken for granted. If high-level disinfection were practiced, the situations suggested here probably would not have occurred or could have been greatly reduced:

- 5,200 Exposed to Hepatitis A from Infected Food Handler

- Continued Salmonella Outbreaks Baffle Health Officials

- 81 Million Americans Exposed Annually to Food-borne Illness Resulting in 7,000 to 8,000 Deaths per year

- 200 Stricken by Contaminated Salad Items in Louisville

- Trench Mouth Reported from Contaminated Glassware

- Fresh Fruits and Vegetables Could be Contaminated with Disease-causing Viruses and Bacteria
- Six Cases of Typhoid, One Case of Salmonella: Shrimp Salad Common to All Victims
- Delaware Shore Dinner Left 150 Ill
- 500 Hit by Salmonella
- Legionnaires Cases Average Two per Week
- Scabies Found on Bedspreads

All of the above outbreaks caused major problems for the people infected and the businesses cited as the source of infection. The consumer is limited to only a few infection-control procedures which will greatly reduce the risk of disease. In a restaurant, wipe off your utensils with a napkin, examine glassware closely, watch how it is carried, be sure your table is free from dirt and food particles, and avoid accepting a meal that has been obviously coughed or sneezed on by a server.

In a hotel or motel room, avoid direct contact with the bedspread, blanket, or head board. Do not touch the telephone mouthpiece with your tongue or lips. Wear foot protection even in the shower.

The hotel, motel, and restaurant establishments one uses for business or pleasure may harbor infectious diseases. Today, the microbiological community is at the most active level of generating new diseases in history. AIDS, Legionnaires, Herpes I and II, and strains of hepatitis are all relatively new diseases within the last 15 years. AIDS is devastating and getting a lot of publicity, but there are still many unanswered questions about the transmission of the virus. Some medical researchers predict a cure will never be found. The common cold is also a viral infection and no cure, after 75 years of research, exists. Hepatitis B is more prevalent than AIDS but gets less media attention. Only after a major disease outbreak occurs is the public informed. Nobody wants to be caught in the wrong place, at the wrong time, and suffer the consequences.

The American Legionnaires Convention in 1976 resulted in loss of lives and the identification of a new bacteria. Legionnaires is still found in evaporative cooling towers, shower heads, and soil. This disease, if not diagnosed and treated, is also fatal.

The diseases present in our environment are transmitted primarily by people or by touching a contaminated surface or object and then rubbing your eye or other natural openings. The public telephone is handled by so many different people it is no wonder that business travelers end up with sore throats or runny noses.

Disease transmission is very likely in hotels, motels, and restaurants, because very few housekeepers, food service workers, or guests wear protective barriers or practice effective personal hygiene. Barriers include disposable gloves and paper towels which can be used to handle glassware or to turn off faucets. Personal hygiene means more than a morning shower or bath; hygiene concerns hair care, hand care, toilet habits, clothing, and so on. Also, most of the chemicals used for sanitizing and disinfecting are either inactive against certain bacteria and viruses or are not used according to the manufacturers' directions. *Sanitize* and *disinfect* are two words that are thought to mean the same thing. However, the food service industry defines sanitize as "free from disease-causing organisms." The microbiological definition of sanitize means only to reduce to a *safe level* the number of microorganisms. A *safe level* is a vague number, based on the number of microorganisms necessary to cause infections and the resistance of the host. Since everybody's resistance levels are different, some people are more susceptible to catching disease.

Defining the terms incorrectly is not the main reason for confusion in the industry. Sanitation products with Environmental Protection Agency (EPA) registration are generally low-to intermediate-level products and would not satisfy the Centers for Disease Control guidelines for health care industry disinfectants. Some *disinfectants* or *sanitizers* only kill Staphylococcus, Salmonella, or Pseudomonas. Certain others kill two out of three bacteria.

There are three levels of disinfection:

- Low–limited level (must kill one gram-negative organism)
- Intermediate–moderate level (must kill two organisms: Staphylococcus and Salmonella)
- High or hospital level (must kill three organisms: Staphylococcus, Salmonella, and Pseudomonas, plus Tuberculosis, pathogenic fungus, and certain specific viruses)

Most household disinfectants are the low to moderate level. This is acceptable in the home, because there is less likelihood of major disease transmission occurrences. However, in businesses serving the public, more attention to disinfection and high-level products should be used.

Microorganisms come in all shapes and sizes; some cause infections easily and others require large quantities or lengthy exposure to transmit a disease.

In today's hustle and bustle, we often tend to overlook the little things and go forward with the *nothing will ever happen to me* attitude. We should be aware of how to reduce the potential spread of infectious diseases. Hotels, motels, and restaurants should be training their employees on how to break the cycle of contamination and how to use high-level disinfection products to supplement cleaning routines. Obviously, with the continued outbreaks of Salmonella, Hepatitis A, and other food-related infections, the industry's standard for sanitation must not be a complete system. Sanitation and personal hygiene are very important, and all hotels, motels, and restaurants emphasize these areas. But do their staffs understand infection control or use high-level disinfection products? Customers paying to enjoy the food and surroundings are entitled to know what is being done to eliminate, or at least greatly reduce, the risk of cross-infection. Here is a list of diseases you can be exposed to in a hotel and/or restaurant:

The common cold
Influenza (flu)
Tuberculosis
Herpes
Staphylococcus infections
Streptococcus infections
Hepatitis
Athletes' foot
Legionnaires
Salmonella
Trench mouth
Intestinal flu
Mononucleosis

Even the virus AIDS has been reported by one researcher to survive outside the host on a surface and to withstand 130° F temperatures for a prolonged period (see Chapter 1). (Transmission of the AIDS virus, however, is still believed to occur primarily through sexual activity and sharing contaminated needles.)

In this book we discuss how these microorganisms can infect you. Consider the following objects found in hotel and motel rooms: sink, toilet, shower/tub, bedspreads, mattress and/or mattress cover, air conditioning system, carpets, furniture, drinking glasses, and telephone. If these surfaces are not effectively disinfected, eliminating any microorganisms that could cause disease, you are at potential risk. Your housekeeper may be an *asymptomatic* (definition: illness or disease present without symptoms or signs of its presence) disease carrier. The previous guest may have had Tuberculosis. Consider that according to microbiologists, 20 percent or more of the population carry some type of infection. Disease-causing microorganisms are found in body fluids, blood, saliva, semen, phlegm, nasal aerosol, body waste, animal waste, *fomites* (definition: any item or object other than food that can propel microorganisms), contaminated food, and contaminated environmental surfaces. The microorganisms continue to mutate, form resistances, and strive for survival just like humans.

A traveler staying in a motel, who had the habit of lounging on top of the bedspread in his underwear, developed a rash and itching shortly after returning home. Upon visiting a doctor, he learned he had picked up scabies, a small parasitic organism that can survive on uncleaned surfaces like bedspreads.

Now, think about your favorite restaurant. The risk to you as a customer comes from contaminated silverware due to inadequate cleaning or sanitizing, contaminated glassware or dinnerware due to exposure from organisms from the hands of employees, air-borne organisms propelled by air-conditioning systems, food contamination from exposure to contaminated environmental surfaces, and/or just the lack of hand washing or barrier protection by food service employees.

I will never eat out again! You do not have to go to that extreme. Hopefully, your favorite eatery practices effective sanitation and personal hygiene or even uses high-level disinfection products to reduce your risk of infection. Examine closely your glassware, silverware, and dinnerware. Wipe your utensils with a napkin or tissue. Watch the way your glasses are carried (from the bottom, not the top), and be sure that nobody sneezes or coughs in your food. Be cautious of restaurants that serve buffet style hors d'oeuvres in the open or use noncooled salad bars. The restaurant can not be responsible for the eating habits of their customers. However, sauces for dipping are always open to cross-contamination from people dipping onto a used saucer, touching the serving implement, and wiping off excess from the saucer back into the large container. Salad bars have similar problems associated with the continued use of serving tongs or utensils constantly touched and dropped back into the large bowls holding the salad items. The food may not have been contaminated when fresh, but an infected customer could be the cause of cross-contamination.

In most cases, the body's normal defenses are strong enough to ward off infections caused by organisms that may be transmitted to restaurant or hotel patrons. If, however, the food handlers or other employees are not practicing infection-control procedures and using the most effective disinfectants available, the risk may still exist. Employee training and new disinfection products are becoming available to the hotel, motel, and restaurant industry. Hopefully, your favorite establishment is utilizing infection-control procedures and products to reduce the risk of cross-contamination. Why not ask on your next visit?

The goals of an infection-control program are simple: reduce the number of microorganisms and break the circle of cross-contamination. These goals can be accomplished without a lot of expense and do not require 20 new people or products to reach the objective. Consumers have the right to information, allowing them to be prepared and more informed about dealing with all businesses. Infections are not limited to hotels, motels, and restaurants, you are at risk in doctors' and dentists' offices, nursing homes, tanning salons, day care centers, work-out spas, and the list goes on.

1

The Need for Infection Control

KEY CONCEPTS

Lifestyle	**Immunity**	**Infection Control**
Public Health	**Resistance**	**OSHA**

In the last 20 to 30 years people have undergone substantial changes in lifestyle in the United States and in other world populations. As a result of these changes, we are living in a much more microbiologically complex world than ever before. New disease transmissions and cross-infection situations are facing the hospitality industry, creating the need for a better understanding of infection control.

World Travel

The United States travel and tourism industry is encouraging international travel, and more Americans are visiting Third

World countries. Many of the Third World nations have virtually no public health facilities or even proper health guidelines. Diseases that are rare in the United States are common in these primitive countries. Thus, Americans traveling to these countries face the risk of cross-infection and ultimately disease. Increased travelers to the United States from the Pacific basin and South America have also opened the door to cross-contamination and the spread of infectious disease from these areas.

The Sex and Drug Revolutions

The sexual revolution and the ready availability of intravenous drugs are among the biggest factors in the increase of the risk of cross-infection. With the prolific use of the Pill in the 1960s, and the growing number of men choosing to have vasectomies, concerns about pregnancy were abated, opening the door to increased sexual activity without fear or consequence. Now media coverage of AIDS, which is theoretically transmitted primarily through sexual intercourse and the use of contaminated needles, has given the phrase "safe sex" a new and deadly connotation.

The Aging of America

The population in the United States is getting older. We are going to have a greater number of elderly people in the 1990s and into the twenty-first century. Aging weakens the immune system and creates greater opportunities for disease transmission. As the numbers of elderly people grow, the impact of all of these factors are magnified.

THE NEED FOR INFECTION CONTROL

It is no longer excusable to ignore potential risk from cross-infection. The Occupational Safety and Health Agency (OSHA) has recently announced its intention to closely monitor the health care professions to ensure that stricter guidelines are observed in order to protect health care workers from the risk of exposure to diseases in the workplace. Penalties for failure to comply to these new regulations result in fines as high as $10,000. OSHA's new surveillance of the health care professions resulted from a failure to implement, on their own, infection-control programs designed to protect both employees and consumers. Government intervention is the result of business and industry's failure to take the initiative of protecting the public and employees.

Public perceptions—and, at this stage, professional estimations—vary widely as to precisely how easily and by what means deadly diseases like AIDS and Hepatitis B can be transmitted to the unwitting public. However, certainly for an industry that prepares and serves food and provides lodging and sanitary facilities to the entire public, the weight of argument over sanitary practices seems to be on the side of caution and conservatism. This is the view of one writer:

> The question of who should disinfect what, how, and where are left unanswered. For example, when an AIDS virus carrier coughs or sneezes secretion into punch bowl or salad bar, the AIDS virus could remain infectious for quite sometime. When a cook or waiter contaminates food with infected saliva or other body fluids, i.e., coughs, sheds infected tears while slicing onions or sustains a cut and contaminates food with blood, what should be done? Should one spray or wash the contaminated foodstuffs with chemical disinfectants? Or should the hapless patron simply swallow hard and hope for the best? In any case, it does appear that a lentivirus which remains infectious for 10

days or longer in a dry form may not be quite as delicate and innocuous outside the body as has been widely rumored [1].

In a study at Mount Sinai Medical Center in Miami Beach, Dr. Lionel Resnick and his co-workers reported finding that the AIDS virus remained infectious for more than a week in liquids at room temperature, and that when dried, it could live 3 days or more [2].*

The study by Resnick suggested that the AIDS virus may not be as weak as it was first thought to be. This does not mean that the virus can be transmitted by casual contact, nor does this endorse the Masters and Johnson theory about AIDS transmission. In a highly controversial book, based on their research, Masters and Johnson suggested that under the right circumstances, the AIDS virus could be transmitted from an environmental surface like a toilet seat. While it still appears that unbroken skin is an effective barrier against the virus, new data are constantly being presented as medical researchers learn more about the virus and it should not be taken for granted. The AIDS virus should be treated with respect and caution should always be taken regarding the possibility of transmission. Since there are so many variables in the areas of concern for lodging and food services, the AIDS virus should be dealt with as highly transmittable and preventive programs and effective disinfection chemicals should be utilized. Hindsight is always 20/20; after disease transmission has occurred, the damage is already done.

Prevention of disease transmission is primarily an exercise in quantity. While it might be highly desirable to eliminate all microorganisms through sterilization, it is not always possible. There are many situations when the best that can be done is disinfecting with the most effective material available. In a cross-infection incident, disease will or will not develop based on the *number* of microorganisms introduced into the host and/or the extent of the host's resistance to disease. The simple concept of reducing the number of organisms to the point where

*Reprinted with permission, Knight-Ridder Newspapers.

the host's immune system can handle the infection naturally should prevent the disease from developing. Consequently, the reduction of microorganisms without complete sterilization can still serve a very useful purpose as part of an infection-control program.

The equation references exactly what occurs with regard to potential disease. If you are healthy and the organism is not virulent, your body's natural defenses can resist the invading organisms. However, if a stronger or more virulent organism enters the body, your defenses may not be capable of warding off the disease. Hepatitis B and AIDS are both virulent organisms.

Prevention of Pathology is a Numbers Game!

$$Health \ vs. \ Disease = \frac{Virulence \times Number \ of \ Organisms}{Resistance \ of \ the \ Host}$$

Hepatitis B

If one cubic centimeter of blood from an infectious carrier of Hepatitis B is mixed with 24,000 gallons of water (relate this to a swimming pool), and one cubic centimeter of this dilution is injected into a susceptible person (anyone without antibodies), there is a 60 to 80 percent likelihood that a serological marker will result.

HIV 1

If one cubic centimeter of blood from an AIDS carrier is placed in one gallon of water and one cubic centimeter of this dilution is injected into a susceptible host, there is a one in ten likelihood of positive infection [3].

It would be advisable for every hospitality establishment to implement some type of infection-control program that is compatible with company policies and objectives before a crisis forces management to play catch-up. It is easier to gradually integrate infection-control procedures without the pressure and stress of deadlines. Crisis management often results in hasty decisions which are not compatible with long-term goals. A program put into effect under the pressure of time does not allow for adequate training of personnel, impedes efficient cost analysis of new products, and, in general, creates disruption of normal operating procedures.

THE MARKETING ADVANTAGE

When a corporation embarks upon an infection-control program, it is very important to include as part of that program a campaign to make consumers aware of the benefits offered.

The food service industry is constantly linked to food- and water-borne disease outbreaks. Environmental agencies which investigate the incidences of illness claim it is nationally recognized that only 5 to 10 percent of the food-related illnesses are reported, and the real number is probably at least 25 times greater than is reported. The Food and Drug Administration feels greater efforts should be made to determine the incidence of all diarrheal and food-borne diarrheal disease. Food-borne diarrheal disease is generally preventable. Prevention is linked directly to infection-control awareness and procedures. In a later chapter, specific transmission examples and numbers will be covered, indicating the types of facility involved, number of people at risk or already ill, and the vehicles of disease transmission.

In the lodging and food service industry, or any other

business, people do not want to admit that mistakes can be made. Marketing is a means for positioning an image. If a hotel or restaurant is linked to a major disease outbreak, the image is negative. By implementing infection-control procedures, training employees, and utilizing high-level disinfection products, a positive image reflecting concern by the property is perceived as positive.

SUMMARY

1. International tourism has contributed to the frequency of disease transmission, partly because many foreign countries do not have public health facilities.

2. Changes in Americans' lifestyles, including increased sexual activities and drug use, have resulted in greater risk of communicable diseases.

3. OSHA is strictly monitoring the implementation of infection control standards in the health care professions, and can be expected to do the same in other occupational settings.

4. AIDS research is constantly providing new information about the virus and its transmission. Meanwhile a careful program of infection control is the only available insurance for the hospitality industry to prevent transmission.

5. It is easier to begin to gradually introduce and implement infection-control procedures now than to be caught unprepared later when such procedures are mandated by the government.

REVIEW EXERCISES

1. In the food service industry only 5 to 10 percent of the related illnesses are reported to local environmental agencies.

    True or False?

2. Today, the microbiological community is in a very active period. Name two new diseases within the last 15 years to have created concern.

    a.

    b.

3. How is disease transmitted most frequently?

    a. contaminated food
    b. people
    c. public telephones
    d. bedspreads

4. How many levels of disinfection exist?

    a. 5
    b. 1
    c. 2
    d. 3

5. A high-level disinfectant must kill

    a. one gram-negative organism like Salmonella
    b. two gram-positive organisms like Streptococcus and Staphylococcus
    c. three organisms, plus Tuberculosis, specific virus, and fungus
    d. Tuberculosis

6. In most cases the body's normal defenses are strong enough to ward off infections.

    True or False?

7. What is the goal of an infection-control program?

2

Fundamentals, Glossary, and Definitions

KEY CONCEPTS

Microbes	**Disinfection**	**Cross-contamination**
Pathogenic	**Transmission**	

The fundamentals of infection control depend upon basic science as it relates to cross-contamination. In order to understand more about infection control and how it relates to the lodging and food service industry, the following definitions, examples of bacteria, and information on modes and routes of transmission are presented.

UNDERSTANDING THE BASICS: A GLOSSARY

The basic terms used in this chapter are presented here as they pertain to the hospitality industry.

Bacteria Living organisms that reproduce.

Virus A small nonliving particle with the capability of entering specific cells, creating changes in the cell and causing it to produce new proteins and additional virus.

Pathogenic Disease-producing.

Aseptic Free of pathogenic bacteria.

Cross-infection Infection passed from one person to another either directly or through contamination of the environment.

Autogenous or **endogenous infection** Infection originating from within one's own body.

Exogenous infection Infection originating from an external source.

Sepsis Presence of pathogenic bacteria; poisonous putrefaction.

Communicable disease A disease capable of being transmitted from person to person.

Mode of transmission Method, device, or vehicle by which microbes are transmitted from one place or organism to another.

Route of transmission Portal, opening, or vehicle through which or by which microbes enter or are carried to the body.

Cutaneous Pertaining to the skin.

Fomite Any article or substance other than food that may transmit pathogenic organisms.

Carrier A person who harbors and disseminates a specific microorganism capable of causing disease in another person. A carrier may be unaffected or may have an invisible or mild case of the disease.

Virulence The relative ease that a microorganism breaks down the body's defenses.

Sterilize Total destruction of all microbial life.

Disinfect Destroy most, but not necessarily all, microorganisms, especially not highly resistant forms such as spores.

Sanitize To make as clean as possible, but not to disinfect.

Sanitize (industry definition) Removal of all disease-causing organisms.

Sanitize (microbiological definition) To reduce to a safe level the number of microorganisms.

MICROBIAL LIFE

Infection control requires a basic working knowledge of microbiology, a somewhat self-explanatory term (*micro* meaning tiny, and *biology* meaning the study of physical life). Microbiology is the study of microorganisms and all factors influencing the life cycle, growth, evolution, function, and death of such organisms.

The human body is engineered to be an ideal host for the growth of microorganisms. Nutrition is supplied to the organisms by blood, serum, decayed food, and other sources, and the normal body temperature of 98.6 degrees Fahrenheit is ideal for rapid growth. Microbes, in fact, play a necessary part in the human life cycle. Without the aid of beneficial microbes in the digestion of food, life would cease. Danger is present only when opportunistic or pathogenic microbes infect the body.

For our purposes, the most important organisms of concern are the pathogenic microbes. These are the disease-causing bacteria and viruses that cause infections. Pathogenic microbes are less abundant than beneficial or nonpathogenic microbes. Some pathogens cause localized infection, such as the common cold; others may affect many different tissues and can be deadly. When your immune system is compromised by a viral infection, the body becomes susceptible to the opportunistic pathogens. These opportunistic microorganisms are normally not harmful, but can detect a break in the body's defenses and become pathogenic.

During a stay in a hotel or motel or during a meal in a restaurant, guests and employees are often exposed to the following kinds of microorganisms:

Gram-Negative Bacteria

Escherichia coli
Pseudomonas species
Aerobacter aerogenes
Salmonella typhosa

Modes of Infection

Unhygienic environments
Carriers
Feces
Hands
Fomites (as defined in the glossary)
Food, water, or milk
Person-to-person contact

Gram-Positive Bacteria

Mycobacterium species (acid-fast)
Staphylococcus aureus
Staphylococcus epidermidi
Streptococcus pyogenes
Bacillus species

Modes of Infection

Person-to-person contact
Nasal and oral secretions
Fomites
Foods
Dust contaminated with living bacillus carriers

Fungi

Aspergillus species
Candida species
Cryptococcus species
Dermatophytes/*Microsporum* species

Modes of Infection

Introduction of fungus into the skin from soil or air contaminates
Mouth/nose/throat
Fomites
Person-to-person contact
Wearing apparel and footwear
Swimming pools or shower stalls
Lockers and floors

Lipophilic Viruses	Modes of Infection
(Viruses having an affinity for fats or other lipides; insoluble in water)	
Influenza	Nasal
Herpes I and II	Sexual contact
	Saliva (possibly)
	Blood

Hydrophilic Viruses	Modes of Infection
(Viruses relating to or having a strong affinity for water; difficult to deactivate)	
Hepatitis	Blood
Poliomyelitis	Saliva
	Nasal droplets

The classification of gram-negative and gram-positive bacteria deals with a means of identifying the bacteria based on its reactions to different staining methods. Gram-negative bacteria are decolorized by alcohol and take a red counterstain. Gram-positive bacteria retain an original stain of violet. Alcohol is one test identification method to categorize bacteria.

Microorganism Update

Bacteria

Actinomyces Gram-positive bacilli resembling fungus.
A. israelli Part of the normal flora of the mouth, throat, and tonsils. Considered to be an opportunistic pathogen.
A. naeslundii Recovered from the human mouth, tonsils, and saliva. Pathogenicity uncertain.
Aeromonas Gram-negative bacilli of the family Pseudomonadaceae

(continued)

A. hydrophila   Occurs in food, lakes, and soil. Causes diarrhea, acute gastroenteritis, arthritis, urinary tract infections, and so on.

Bacillus   Gram-positive spore-forming rod.

B. cereus   Widely distributed in dust, soil, milk, and on plants. Associated with food poisoning.

Borrelia and *Treponema*   Gram-negative microorganisms.

B. buccuals and B. vincentii; T. buccale and T. vincentii   Isolated from the gums in normal mouths and mucous membranes of the respiratory tract. Associated with "trench mouth."

Diplococcus pneumoniae   A gram-positive encapsulated *Diplococcus* from the *Streptococceae*; 38 to 70 percent of the population carries this organism. Common cause of bacterial pneumonia. Also causes conjunctivitis, peritonitis, sinusitis, and so on.

Enterococci   Part of the normal flora of the intestines, but may cause disease when transferred from the intestinal habitat into the blood stream. Occasionally, associated with food poisoning. Susceptibility to drugs vary widely.

Erysipelothrix rhusiopathiae   Present worldwide. Causes skin infections from contact of infected materials (meat, fish, poultry, manure, hides, and bones).

Escherichia   Widely distributed in nature and in the human intestinal tract.

E. coli   Causes urinary tract infections, wound infections, summer diarrhea, diarrhea of travelers, especially to Mexico, Central and South America, Europe, and Asia.

Leptospira   Humans acquire infection from ingestion of sources such as rats, mice, cattle, horses, hogs, goats, dogs, and wild rodents. Many infections are subclinical (invisible).

(continued)

Pseudomonas Gram-negative rods widely distributed in nature in soil, water, air, and sewage.

P. alcaligenes Found in raw milk, swimming pools, frozen fish, and feces. Causes infections of urinary tract, respiratory system, and so on.

Salmonella All *Salmonella* species (except *S. typhi*) are contracted orally by transmission from contaminated milk and water, and such foods as eggs, ice cream, meringue pies, shellfish, and undercooked chicken, fish, or pork.

S. arizonae Causes acute diarrhea from contaminated food.

S. derby Responsible for food poisoning or gastrointestinal type of illness.

S. gallinarum Produces food poisoning and so on.

S. typhimurium Frequently causes food poisoning and so on.

Staphylococcus Common in the air and environment; some are considered to be a part of the normal flora of the skin. Because of the great number of resistant strains, all infections require antimicrobial susceptibility test.

S. aureus Food poisoning, produces pimples, abscesses, and so on.

Streptococcus Widely distributed in water, dust, vegetation, milk, and dairy products. Capable of producing disease in almost every organ of humans.

Group C *Streptococci* Has been isolated from the respiratory tract of humans. Occasionally, responsible for epidemic sore throat through ingestion of contaminated milk.

Group D *Streptococci* Isolated from humans, animals, and milk. May cause subacute bacterial endocarditis and urinary tract and wound infections.

Group F *Streptococci* Has been isolated most com-

(continued)

monly from the human throat and has been associated with tonsillitis.

Group G *Streptococci* (*S. anginosus*) Has been isolated from the throat, nose, feces, vagina, and skin and has been implicated in respiratory infections.

Group H *Streptococci* (*S. sanguis*) Has been isolated from the respiratory tract of humans.

Group N *Streptococci* Includes *S. lactis,* frequently present in milk and *S. cremoris,* found in cream. Causes milk souring.

Fungi

Aspergillus A genus of approximately 300 fungal species which are ubiquitous. The spores are air borne. Causes skin lesions, conjunctivitis, eye infections, and so on.

Candida Yeastlike fungi, can cause candidiasis.

C. krusei Isolated from skin, beer, and milk products.

C. pseudotropicalis Isolated from nail infections. Also, found in cheese and dairy products.

Microsporum A genus of dermatophytic fungi that may infect hair or skin and cause *tinea corporis, tinea barbae, tinea capitis,* and *tinea favosa*. Found worldwide.

Phialophora Commonly present in soil, decaying wood, and water and on fruit and vegetables. Many species.

Trichophyton May cause infections of the hair, skin, nails, and so on.

T. megninii Skin lesions of the hand, foot, and beard areas. Primarily in Europe.

T. metagrophytes Causes ectothrix infections, chronic Athletes' foot, and skin lesions.

T. pedis Athletes' foot. 50 to 90 percent of the population is affected at some time in their lives [4].

MODES AND ROUTES OF TRANSMISSION

The body provides a natural resistance to microbial invasion. It is only when these defense systems are broken down or cut that the body is exposed to infection. In order to understand the transmission of disease from one person to another, from a person to an object, or from an object to a person, we must remember the basic principles of how the human body works.

To begin with, the body constantly sheds old and dead cells, in order to regenerate new cells. The main factor here is dead skin slough as well as hair. It is estimated that the average adult sheds millions of cells—approximately two and a half million from the hands alone—and 80 to 100 hairs daily. The favored hand, right or left, has over 100 microscopic openings which can allow for the transmission of disease. Add to this the fact that all microorganisms are hitchhikers that have no means of propulsion and therefore, ride upon particulate matter (skin slough, hair, moisture particles, or dust) and eventually settle on surfaces or food where they can be picked up or ingested. Hence, a lodging establishment possesses all the elements conducive to possible transmission of organisms and needs to establish a proper infection-control program to minimize the risk and impact of viral or bacteriological diseases. All personnel should be made aware of the part they play in safeguarding customers and other staff members.

Cross-contamination

The question is frequently asked, "Are hotels, motels, and restaurants really a source of cross-contamination?" There has been no formal study, but it is logical that exposure does occur and that employees and guests are vulnerable. There are medical and dental procedures that take place in hospitals, nursing homes, and other institutions which overlap some of the basic housekeeping and food preparation steps routinely performed on a daily basis, and these indicate a more than positive parallel for cross-contamination. It was reported in April 1987 [5]* and July 1987 [6]** that Hepatitis A outbreaks occurred and were traced to food handlers. In early 1988, additional outbreaks of Hepatitis A linked to food were reported [7]. Other cases of Salmonella continue to baffle health officials.

A typical example of cross-contamination involves the contact between a food handler–carrier harboring a disease such as hepatitis and an unsuspecting customer. The food handler nicks his or her finger while preparing a salad and, since no hand protection is being worn and no antimicrobial soap has been used, this exposure allows the hepatitis virus to enter the customer's system, food being the mode of transmission.

In another scenario, a salesman returns to his room to relax prior to dinner or additional meetings with clients. The guest lies on top of the bedspread in his underwear and, due to lack of proper disinfection of the bedspread, takes home scabies. Scabies is a small microorganism that causes constant itching and a rash [8]. This person and his entire family must undergo thorough disinfecting procedures, getting rid of the organism. This could have been prevented by the application of a disinfectant product to the bedspread that would break the cycle of infection/contamination and eliminate cross-contamination.

*Reprinted with permission from The Seattle Times.
**Copyright © 1987 by The New York Times Company. Reprinted by permission.

Routes of Transmission/Portals of Disease Entry

Oral: swallow
Percutaneously: intact skin penetrated by needle,
    knife, etc.
Inhaled: respiratory

(continued)

Eyes: open moist orifice; exposure to mucous membrane

Sexual: genitals, anal: exposure to mucous membrane

Ear: open orifice: exposure to mucous membrane

Lesion: from dermatitis, break in the skin via nicks, cuts, scratches, and so on.

Cell slough: the human body sloughs two and a half million cells a day from the hands alone.

Infectious Diseases: A Nationwide Concern

Legal responsibility:

It is the legal responsibility of employers to provide appropriate safeguards....

As enforced by OSHA
Source: Federal Register

Diseases Potentially Transmitted in a Room Environment

Cold

Flu

Tuberculosis

Herpes

Staphylococcus Infections

Streptococcus Infections

Hepatitis

Athletes' Foot

Legionnaires' Disease

Diseases Potentially Transmitted in a Food Service Environment to the Customer

Salmonella
Hepatitis A
Staphylococcus
Streptococcus
Herpes
Trench Mouth
Intestinal Flu

Risk Situations in Which Disease Can Be Transmitted in a Housekeeping Function to an Employee

Moist towels
Body fluids on environmental surfaces, toilet seats, sink,
    sheets, tub, shower
Bed wetter
Vomit
Soap soup
Air-conditioning systems
Accumulations of air-borne organisms on surface, drapes,
    bedspreads

Risk to Guests from Room Occupancy

Sink
Toilet
Telephone
Mattress
Air conditioner

(continued)

Tub/shower
Carpet
Drinking glasses
Towels, washcloths, laundry

Risk of Disease Transmission to Food Service Employees

Sharp utensils—nicks, cuts, and so on.
Handling silverware, glasses, and so on, after use by customer.
Burns
Bar soap
Common towels
Risk of cross-contamination of an open lesion, wound or abrasion from environmental surfaces
Slippery surfaces
Transmission through uncleaned foods (such as lettuce)

Contamination and Exposure Risks to Guests

Contaminated silverware due to inadequate cleaning or sanitizing
Contaminated glassware or dinnerware due to exposure from organisms from the hands of employees
Exposure to air-borne organisms on tables, counters, etc., promoted by air-conditioning systems
Hepatitis risk from infected food handlers
Food contamination from exposure to contaminated environmental surfaces
Poor or nonexistent hand washing and failure to use antimicrobial soaps
Failure to use barrier protection by employees

SUMMARY

1. Microbial life is all around us. Some microorganisms are necessary for survival; others can cause many types of infections.

2. Hotels, motels, and restaurants are exposed to disease-causing microorganisms.

3. Food poisoning and other potential infections can occur in our properties.

REVIEW EXERCISES

1. Disease producing microorganisms are:
   a. pathogens
   b. carriers
   c. spores

2. The process of passing infection from one person to another is:
   a. cross-contamination
   b. endogenous infection
   c. carrier contamination

3. Modes of microorganism transmission include:
   a. blood
   b. saliva
   c. semen
   d. all of the above
   e. b and c

4. To make an environment as clean as possible, but not to disinfect it is to:
   a. sanitize

    b. septicize

    c. sterilize

5. A goal of an infection-control program is:

    a. to get new customers

    b. to sterilize

    c. to reduce the number of microbes in the environment

6 Some microorganisms have their own means of propulsion:

True or False?

7. The human body can exist without microorganisms:

True or False?

8. Nonpathogenic microbes are more abundant than pathogenic microbes:

True or False?

9. Autogenous (a) or Exogenous (b) infection originates from outside the body:

a or b?

Relevant Diseases

KEY CONCEPTS

Hepatitis   **AIDS**   **Herpes**
Legionnella   **Tuberculosis**   **Salmonella Poisoning**

On a daily basis, large numbers of pathogenic organisms may be carried into and out of hotels, motels, and restaurants by customers, travelers, employees, and delivery people.

Listed below are some of the diseases which under the right circumstances, are known or suspected to be transmittable in a lodging and hospitality setting. Some of these will be discussed in this chapter.

Some diseases are more serious threats because they have fewer warning signs. Employees should, therefore, be strongly motivated at all times to protect themselves and others from cross-infection.

Diseases in some cases become controlled or are eliminated; other new diseases are discovered or old ones evolve and become more serious. We once thought we had tuberculosis under control, only to realize that the disease is on the increase among the homeless, nursing home patients, and AIDS victims. Obviously, there is still a lot more research to be done on infectious diseases. The microbiological community is ever active and continues to create a challenge for medical and viral and bacteriological research.

A researcher summarizing problems with AIDS and other diseases stated [9]:

> Microbes, which have existed on this planet far longer than man, show no signs of being unconditionally conquered. Amid the billions that exist harmoniously around us, there will always be some that become unexpectedly disruptive, mysteriously virulent.

Remember that microbes and viruses mutate, change, and evolve and like all life forms, strive for survival!

HEPATITIS

Hepatitis in all of its four forms (A, B, C or Non-A, and Non-B and D) is a viral infection of the liver. Hepatitis B, some types of Hepatitis C, and Hepatitis D are primarily associated with certain lifestyles involving intravenous drug abuse and promiscuous sexual activity, particularly homosexual, but can also be transmitted through contaminated medical instruments or in blood transfusions.

Hepatitis B, C, and D have long incubation periods and carrier status may last for a lifetime. Hepatitis B is particularly infectious and virulent. According to the Centers for Disease Control, in a cubic centimeter of blood from a Hepatitis B carrier there are 100 million virus. As little as one-millionth of a cubic centimeter of blood from a carrier can transmit a clinical case of Hepatitis B.

In the United States, an estimated 300,000 new cases of Hepatitis B per year are reported. Currently, there are approximately two million carriers, and the pool grows yearly. Health authorities estimate that there are 3,000 dentists and auxiliary personnel who are carriers [10].

Hepatitis A is transmitted in the lodging and food service context through contaminated food or beverages, via water containing human waste, or by infected food handlers. In major metropolitan areas, as much as 10 to 15 percent of the population may have been exposed to Hepatitis A.

The hospitality industry was linked to approximately 300 cases of Hepatitis A transmission through the first eight months of 1987 alone [5,6]. One outbreak in 1988 on the West Coast, which affected over 3,000 people, was traced to an infected food handler [11].

The Centers for Disease Control estimate that over one million cases of Hepatitis B occur annually but only 200,000 to 300,000 cases are reported due to the fact that the other 80 percent are subclinical or invisible cases and not readily detected. Some carriers may transmit the Hepatitis B virus for years and still not be aware they have or carry the disease.

Even though Hepatitis B is preventable by a vaccine, the disease continues to spread. It is also important to note that Hepatitis B is much more prevalent outside the United States in Third World countries. This means that due to the many possibilities of transmission by contact from blood, saliva, or other body fluids, travelers are constantly vulnerable to infection. Hepatitis B and other identified types of hepatitis pose an ongoing threat because more people are at risk and the disease is very virulent. It is recommended in situations where a definite risk to exposure exists that the vaccine be administered.

Hepatitis is one of the diseases that must be reported to the Centers for Disease Control. Many others that cause severe problems may not be as newsworthy, but can still devastate the reputation of a business.

Hepatitis A, as well as other strains, should be of great concern to lodging and hospitality businesses because currently no infection-control procedures or products are utilized on a daily basis to prevent cross-contamination.

LEGIONNELLOSIS (LEGIONNAIRES' DISEASE)

Legionnella is a bacterium that attacks the respiratory system. Primarily, it targets men who are approximately 55 years of age, overweight, and smokers. It is usually found in evaporative air-conditioning systems, and once inhaled, it can be fatal. It has a two to three week incubation period and is fatal if not treated in time.

Legionnella pneumophila A very small gram-negative, aerobic bacilli found in streams and air-conditioning cooling water [12].

Broad Street pneumonia A respiratory illness that may occur sporadically or in epidemics, predominantly in late summer and early fall.

In July and August 1976, an outbreak of febrile respiratory illness resulting in deaths occurred in Philadelphia, Pennsylvania [13]. The hotel property that hosted the American Legion Convention that summer is still suffering from the repercussions. It is important to note that this was not the first documented outbreak now believed to have been caused by the Legionnaires' disease bacterium. In 1974, the same hotel property experienced two deaths in another group's convention.

Legionnaires' disease has not disappeared; an average of two cases a week are reported to the Centers for Disease Control.

In July of 1985, a sales associate of the J. D. Group, Infection Control Consultants, was diagnosed with Legionnaires' disease. In tracing his travels, a hotel in Nebraska was the probable source. When the general manager was contacted, his first concern was about being sued; his second was about getting board approval to take action. As far as anyone knows the problem may still exist in the cooling system of that property.

It is important to remember that the Legionnaires' disease bacterium is transmitted through the air. The environmental sources implicated are cooling tower water associated with air-conditioning systems and soils broken up by construction work and transported by air currents. Not only are evaporative cooling systems a concern, therefore, but new construction still spreads the bacteria from newly broken soil. Wouldn't a group of investors or a major corporation building a new facility be horrified if Legionnaires' disease bacterium caused illness resulting in the loss of millions of dollars because no one had the foresight to have soil and water analyzed prior to construction?

HERPES SIMPLEX I AND II

This emerging disease affects the lifestyle of more than the rich and famous. It is estimated that there are five million cases of Herpes II in the United States alone. Primarily considered a venereal disease, Herpes II is devastating to its victims. Outbreaks can occur five to eight times per year. Symptoms include lesions, extreme pain, fever, genital discharge, and general malaise. Lesions occur on the genital area, buttocks, fingers, thighs, and occasionally other parts of the body.

Herpes II is mainly transmitted by sexual contact and the passing of body fluids. The effects of this viral disease, as well as those of Herpes I, oral Herpes, can be traumatic and possibly affect job performance.

Herpes Simplex I, or HSV, causes a variety of illnesses. Infections may result from people whose immune systems are compromised, spread from customers to employees, and employees to customers. HSV infections are spread by direct contact and oral secretions. A common characteristic of the virus is their ability to persist, generally in latent infection, in cells of a host.

Preventive measures for employees include avoiding direct contact with open lesions, cuts, or burns, wearing hand protection, and thorough hand washing after any possible exposure.

Herpes Simplex I is more abundant than Herpes Simplex II but due to the variety of Herpes viruses it is difficult to treat and cure some of them. Herpes Simplex II is incurable, but can be treated with salves, creams, and ointments to reduce the pain. Herpes is just one of the over 50 sexually transmitted diseases we currently deal with in our society. Persons who suspect they may have had contact with an infected person who has a sexually transmitted disease, or persons experiencing symptoms such as discharge, sores, or rash, should seek prompt medical attention.

AIDS

The media have increased public awareness about Acquired Immune Deficiency Syndrome (AIDS). In 1987 alone over 20,000 new cases were diagnosed in the United States. World-wide, nearly 140,000 cases were reported in 1988. The World Health Organization estimated the real number of adult cases was between 350,000 and 400,000 for all of 1988. It remains to be seen, therefore, how many more cases will be reported as this virus continues to devastate humanity. A 1989 study by the Hudson Institute in Washington, D.C., predicted a "worst-case" scenario of 14.5 million Americans infected by the year 2002, unless major changes take place in social–sexual attitudes and a vaccine is developed. AIDS is a blood-borne virus transmitted primarily via sexual contact, contaminated intravenous needles, or blood. The incubation period is from one year up.

AIDS was first observed in homosexual men, drug users, and hemophiliacs. Heterosexual incidents of transmission have spread the disease beyond the original pool to the so-called "straight" community, averaging 4 percent of all cases. The Centers for Disease Control do not fully breakdown all the data revealing specific categories based on the multiple risks that exist. For example, there may be homosexual drug users that are only classified in the homosexual grouping. The 4 percent estimate of heterosexual incident in the best judgement of the author pertains to non-homosexual non-drug users. If the drug users were included in the percentage, it would be higher. This is predicted by the Centers for Disease Control possibly to climb to 7 percent.

The classic AIDS infection attacks specific cells in the immune system resulting in the death of those cells and rendering the immune system inoperable. The primary age group is from 20 to 49 years in all racial and ethnic groups. Symptoms begin like the common cold, with fever, sweats, and swollen glands, then progress to consistent weight loss, diarrhea, persistent cough, general malaise and weakness, and occasionally a purplish colored rash. Figure 3.1 shows a normal immune system with the T helper (TH) cells outnumbering the T suppressor (TS) cells generating natural defenses to fight off infection. Figure 3.2 shows the 2:1 ratio reversed TS cells to TH cells not allowing the immune system to function properly.

Most health authorities involved with AIDS research or AIDS patient treatment recognize three stages of the AIDS syndrome:

In Stage I, the individual has been infected with the virus and antibodies have developed, but the host is unaffected symptomatically by the virus. The immune system remains intact and functional, and the health of the host seems unchanged. This condition can remain indefinitely. During this phase the host is asymptomatic but can transmit the disease to others with whom he or she has intimate contact or who are exposed to his or her blood or other body fluids. The Centers for Disease Control estimate that there are between two and three million asymptomatic carriers of the AIDS virus.

During Stage II, the host begins to experience some of the opportunistic diseases which may ultimately prove fatal. These diseases are either rare among the general population or are normally treated with relative ease. However, with a compromised immune system, these diseases persist. The individual in Stage II can usually still function, but requires considerable medical support.

In Stage III, the opportunistic diseases overwhelm the host despite any medical efforts. The longest known survival period in Stage III is about 58 weeks. No research so far, despite the $1.2 billion budget from the government, has produced anything closely resembling a cure. One recent concern expressed by the Centers for Disease Control is that the transmission of the disease may be more closely linked to environmental factors than was previously thought. This is

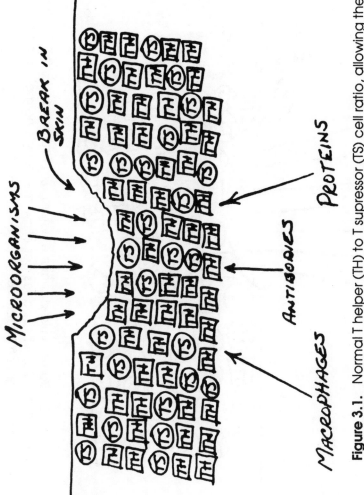

Figure 3.1. Normal T helper (TH) to T supressor (TS) cell ratio, allowing the body's immune system to produce macrophages, antibodies, and protein to ward off infections. (Drawing compliments of Mr. Richard Yobel.)

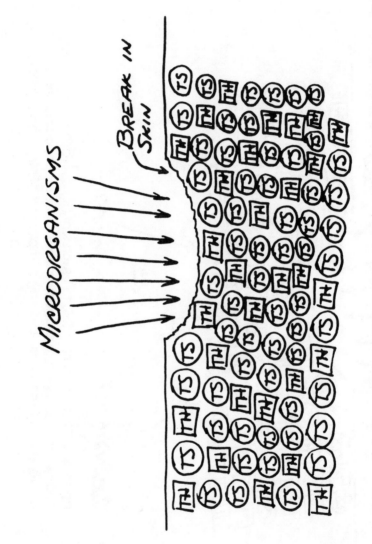

Figure 3.2. Compromised immune system with T supressor (TS) in 2:1 ratio over T helper (TH) cells, which does not allow the body's normal defences to work properly to fight off infections.

based on the fact that in the United States the heterosexual transmission experienced in the African model has not materialized, leading some observers to look for an environmental link in the chain of AIDS transmission.

Estimates vary between 5 and 15 percent as to the number of asymptomatic carriers who will progress from Stage I to Stage III. It is impossible to predict which individuals will be so afflicted, but co-factor diseases appear to have some effect. This simply means that if a carrier is afflicted with a subsequent infection such as hepatitis, herpes, or other infections, the immune system becomes stimulated and more damage can be sustained.

Until further evidence is available, the most conservative assumption for the lodging and hospitality industry must be that AIDS, under the right circumstances, could be transmitted by exposure to the virus on environmental surfaces or eating utensils.

SALMONELLA

In the food service industry, constant attention is given to food-borne illness. Food will never be totally disinfected, sterilized, or free from bacteria and potential contaminants. Current sanitation and health standards very clearly address the proper receiving, storage, handling, and preparation of food. Unfortunately, somewhere in route from processors to customer an error can allow the transmission of a bacterium. Salmonella infections are a major contributor to the millions of Americans exposed to contaminated food. Food-borne illness accounts for over 8,000 deaths a year. Salmonella incubate for 6 to 48 hours, can last 2 to 3 days, and cause stomach pain, fever, vomiting, diarrhea, and headaches, a very unpleasant experience. It generally comes from meats, poultry, and protein foods or food handler carriers. Contaminated food must be prepared properly and not held for longer than the recommended 2 hours at the appropriate cooking and storing temperatures. The lack of personal hygiene and improper hand washing or uncleanliness is inexcusable. In the meantime, Salmonella continues to cause infections and generate problems for the food service industry.

Other bacteria specifically relative to food-borne illness can be reviewed in *Applied Foodservice Sanitation* by the Educational Foundation of the National Restaurant Association [14].

TUBERCULOSIS

Tuberculosis, predominantly a respiratory disease, is not only limited to the lungs, and can strike other organs of the body as well.

In 1987, based on the Centers for Disease Control reports, tuberculosis increased 2 percent above normal outbreaks. A main reason was due to the opportunistic pneumocystis carinii pneumonia or PCP, a parasitic form of pneumonia that attacks AIDS victims. This reinforces the fact that the old diseases once thought controlled or subsided are still a part of the microbiological community. The new diseases caused by new viruses and bacteria must be addressed, and the risk of infection reduced. This requires an awareness of state-of-the-art high-level disinfection and infection-control procedures for all concerned.

THE IMPORTANCE OF INFECTION CONTROL TO EMPLOYERS AND EMPLOYEES

The major goal of an effective infection-control program is to prevent cross-contamination, thereby protecting all guests and personnel from acquiring a serious or fatal disease.

The constant movement of employees, travelers, and customers has opened the door to potential litigation. Obviously, the public is becoming more concerned about specific rights, if involved in some type of litigation. More lawyers are advertising contingent fees or no fees unless settlement is reached, making law suits more attractive and making businesses that are negligent more vulnerable. Being negligent simply means that if in some way prevention was possible and not practiced or steps were not taken to ensure the safety of all concerned, the door is open for a liability suit.

The second purpose of an infection-control program is to protect properties from shutdown or loss of revenue.

Another goal of an infection-control protocol is making sure all proper testing is performed as prevention before an outbreak can occur. Action instead of reaction or prevention instead of a problem are models of preparation.

The following information on the transmission of disease and how it specifically relates to lodging and food service employees or guests, will emphasize why proper testing or preventive measures should be taken to greatly reduce the possibility of cross-contamination. The specific risk situations identify breeding places for disease-causing organisms and the types of illnesses and infections which can come from specific bacteria and viruses which can, under the right circumstances, be transmitted from employee to guest or guest to employee or from the environmental surfaces to both employees and guests.

Infectious diseases are present in our daily activities and must be properly addressed to reduce the potential for liabilities and create a safer healthier environment in which to reside. The Centers for Disease Control are still identifying new viruses and bacteria. Most are harmless, but, for example, in one recent instance, an upstate New York property was closed because of an unidentified organism that was somehow passed along to a guest. In the event that a viral or bacteriological disease is definitely linked to a hotel, motel, or restaurant, the property may end up being closed. Even if it is not closed, once the public becomes aware of the problem, the damage to business may be irreparable. In many metropolitan areas, local newspapers publish notices of the closing of establishments connected with food-borne or other disease transmission.

We all have the right to expect the highest standards of service, based on the standards that ensure a healthier safer environment in which to live and work. If no standards exist, or if effective programs are not implemented, there will be less of a need for hospitality and fewer worries about our personnel pool and how to attract new revenues.

SUMMARY

1. All people are exposed to disease-causing microorganisms.
2. No work environment is completely free from potentially infectious organisms.
3. AIDS is definitely a serious new disease; however, hepatitis also having many asymptomatic carriers, is far more infectious and afflicts far more people annually.
4. Disease can be spread by blood, bodily fluids, and other normal routes of transmission. After entering the body some microbes can damage the natural cell reproduction system, creating irreversible damage.

REVIEW EXERCISES

1. Food service and lodging personnel are potentially exposed to:
   a. many virulent diseases

    b. an occasional infection

    c. a large number of pathogens

2. Name three serious diseases found in the workplace:

    a.

    b.

    c.

3. Whenever a particular disease is conquered:

    a. it is controlled indefinitely

    b. the survival age increases

    c. others evolve to seriousness

4. The most serious emerging disease is:

    a. AIDS

    b. hepatitis

    c. Legionnaires

5. A common route of transmission of Hepatitis B is:

    a. saliva

    b. blood

    c. cut on finger

6. An effective infection-control program will automatically cope with:

    a. AIDS

    b. herpes

    c. hepatitis

7. Which is the most virulent form of hepatitis?

    a. A

    b. B

    c. C

    d. D

8. Which bodily system does AIDS attack?

    a. circulatory

    b. digestive

    c. immune

    d. reproductive

9. What is the normal ratio of T helper cells and T suppressor cells in a healthy immune system?

10. What natural defenses does the normal ratio of TH to TS cells allow the body's immune system to produce? Name two.

    a.

    b.

4

The Employee and Infection Control

KEY CONCEPTS

Hygiene	**Sepsis**	**Asepsis**
Screening		

In the past, customers and travelers have selected a place to stay or eat based on the following factors:

1. Business needs
2. Vacation objectives
3. Atmosphere
4. Convenience
5. Cost
6. Cuisine
7. Location
8. Special services and athletic facilities

In general, infection control has not been a major factor in the selection of a lodging or eating establishment. However, today's travelers are more aware of infectious diseases due to media coverage of food poisoning, Legionnaires' disease, AIDS, and other serious disease outbreaks.

Flight attendants on airplanes have been overheard discussing whether handling airsick travelers is safe. Customers in restaurants are examining their utensils more closely for cleanliness and making sure no smudges or stains appear on glassware. This increased consumer and employee awareness mandates that the lodging and hospitality industry address the issue of infection control.

Within the industry, the second most important consideration—after the implementation of an effective infection-control program based on appropriate guidelines from recommended authorities—is the hiring, training, and motivation of competent personnel.

Since at the entry level of employment there is a great deal of turnover, and since infection control is a continuous learning process, ongoing programs are necessary to encourage the management staff to get involved and to formalize standard procedures which all employees can easily follow.

Personal Care and Hygiene

Customer protection begins with personal care and hygiene of each staff member.

CLOTHING

Proper staff dress is important to a well-rounded infection-control program. If uniforms are worn by housekeeping and restaurant personnel, they should be simple, as seamless as possible, and have short sleeves. Studies have shown that microorganisms accumulate on the cuffs of long-sleeved uniforms. Specific studies have been done by the dental profession on uniforms worn by auxiliary personnel. Similar conclusions could be made about any long-sleeve or cotton uniforms worn by housekeepers or food service personnel. The simple test of touching the surface of a uniform with a rodac plate and culturing the plate for 24 hours, would reveal dramatic evidence of fabric contamination.

The uniform should withstand frequent and multiple washings. Synthetic materials retain fewer microbes and are sturdier than cotton. When possible, uniforms should be kept on the premises; personnel wearing their uniforms while commuting by public transportation, or even in private vehicles, can soil or contaminate a fresh uniform. It doesn't make sense to properly disinfect work surfaces and other countertops and at the same time wear contaminated clothing.

Hair Care

All personnel should have short manageable hair; long hair should be kept restrained or covered.

HAND WASHING

All employees, regardless of work assignments, should wash their hands frequently. Hands should be washed even if disposable gloves are worn. The University of Georgia College of

Agriculture [15] has studied hand washing extensively, and the results of their work emphasizes the values of multiple washings and the use of antimicrobial sanitizing soap. Fingernails should be kept short and clean and should never be cleaned with a sharp, pointed object, which could break the skin under the nail. It has been shown that many pathogens can be protected for many days under fingernails. Artificial fingernails are not recommended.

Hand Washing Technique

An acceptable hand washing technique in conjunction with an antimicrobial soap requires only 30 to 45 seconds. The soap should be applied and rubbed over the hands and wrists and then rinsed off with warm water. The second soap application should be more rigorously rubbed and rinsed. Using this double application technique, with the first application slightly heavier on soap than on water and the second soap application and scrubbing procedure immediately following, provides a quick and safe way of protecting the hands.

In most cases all guest room baths are equipped with standard hand-actuated faucets. These should be disinfected between guests. Restroom facilities should be disinfected frequently. Employees should always use disposable paper towels to dry their hands and should use the towel to turn off the faucet. The towel will serve as a protective barrier, avoiding contamination from the faucet.

All soap and lotion dispensers used by employees should be wall-hung or foot-actuated. Hot air dryers are recommended. Cloth towels should not be used unless absolutely necessary, and they should only be used once.

SCREENING FOR RISK

Unfortunately, there is no way of avoiding risk by screening the guests who check in or order a meal. Any precaution taken or disinfectant product effectively introduced into the environment, therefore, can help to reduce the possibility of cross-contamination.

Hotel, motel, or restaurant managers may wish to ask as part of the screening process for all entry-level employees, very specific questions pertaining to disease.

Since most medical questions are very technical and often difficult to understand, the J.D. Group, Inc. has designed an Employee Health Form and assigned a point scoring system to provide the employer with enough information to recommend a physical examination be taken by a job candidate to identify if a real risk situation exists. The questions have been compiled based on researching various types of health questions used by doctors and dentists. We include a sample of this form here (see pages 54–55).

These questions must be asked of all employees to avoid discrimination difficulties. Such questions are primarily designed to be used in dental offices where patients are asked to give a brief medical history. These questions are specifically designed to see if patients have been or are carriers of Hepatitis B. The blood test questions and question #5 are asked because, as we discussed, Hepatitis B is a very virulent disease and capable of transmission from more casual exposure.

Since doctors and dentists have the advantage of taking medical histories from new patients and then upon examination can by blood test or other methods detect if an infection or illness exists, a similar form should be part of a new employee's file. Generally, persons responsible for hiring new employees are not trained to detect disease carriers. Since in many cases new employees are hired off the streets, a need for better awareness about disease dictates improved screening of employees to better determine the current status of their health.

Since the federal government has outlined that no employee shall work in a capacity in which there is a likelihood of that employee contaminating food, utensils, or food contact surfaces or working with external lesions unless properly covered, and has classified AIDS carriers as handicapped as covered under the right to work and equal opportunity employment act, the need for more medical information about the health and well being of the prospective employee would seem essential. If no guidelines or questions are recommended and an asymptomatic disease carrier is hired and then transmits a disease to other employees or customers, the property is liable. Civil rights are important to everyone and are not meant to be challenged by asking questions about one's health for the purpose of determining if problems which may need medical treatment exist.

Employee Health Form

1. Have you been under the care of a physician in the last 12 months?
2. Have you experienced any health problems or illness that has lasted longer than 1 month and kept you from working?
3. Have you had a surgical procedure (operation) in the last two years?
4. Have you ever received a blood transfusion?
5. Have you ever had yellowed skin and white of the eyes or a liver infection?
6. Have you ever been identified by a physician as a carrier of any contagious disease, even though you were not sick?

(continued)

---

7. Have you ever received treatment for substance abuse?
8. Have you ever experienced an allergic reaction to any drug or medication?
9. Have you ever experienced any of the following:
    a. Unexplained weight loss
    b. Night sweats
    c. Swollen glands
    d. Prolonged diarrhea
10. Have you ever traveled outside of the United States? If yes, state how long and give the location.
11. Do you have any type of skin disorder or dermatitis?

Point Evaluation System

If the employee responds with a yes answer, the following points are assigned to each question:
1. 1 point, if yes
2. 2 points
3. 1 point
4. 3 points
5. 2 points
6. 4 points
7. 4 points
8. 1 point
9. 2 points for each yes answer
10. 2 points for the Mid-East or Far East
    1 point for Canada or Western Europe
11. 2 points

Total points: 25
  Over 15 points—medical alert
  Over 18 points—require a physical
  Over 20 points—probable contagious disease
                    carrier

The Employee Health Form is designed to be used as a tool to help the employer identify potential contagious disease risks. The employer is then able to establish where this possible high-risk employee is best suited to work. If the property has an infection-control protocol established, which identifies precautions to be observed by all workers, outlining specific barrier protection and other infection-control guidelines, it is advisable to share this information during the personnel interview along with the health form.

The public awareness level makes even the smallest effort by our industry beneficial to the well being of all our employees and guests.

High-Risk Employee Precautions

When it is discovered that an employee either fits into a defined high-risk group or shows outward symptoms of a communicable disease, good aseptic techniques will minimize the potential of disease transmission.

1. The employee should be requested to wear disposable latex gloves, an apron and/or other additional protective barriers, a disposable cap, mask, and so on.
2. If the employee will be working in a food service area, a disposable mask should be required in addition to gloves and apron.
3. All surfaces in the work area should be disinfected daily.
4. All employees should wash their hands frequently with an antimicrobial soap.
5. Care should be taken to avoid nicks, cuts, or other job-related skin irritations. If they occur, gloves should be worn constantly.

(continued)

6. Cloth towels should not be used in food service or bathroom areas for personal purposes.
7. Hair should be short or restrained and covered properly.
8. Fingernails should be short. Artificial nails are not recommended.
9. In case of contamination of work surfaces by blood or other fluids, the surface should be cleaned and disinfected immediately.
10. Employees should fill out employee health forms and update them periodically.
11. Culture sampling from surfaces in food service and housekeeping areas should be done routinely to identify any needs for special infection-control procedures.
12. Make sure all employees are aware of and have proper instruction regarding infection-control products and procedures that are in place.

Even in a clean guest room or a clean kitchen area, sepsis (the presence of microorganisms in large quantities) still exists. This is because most of the products used for cleaning may remove or eliminate some microorganisms, but many organisms have formed a resistance to the once effective sanitation chemicals and still thrive. The continuum shown on page 58 lists procedures that cover the levels of clean from sepsis to asepsis.

The purpose of the continuum is to offer suggestions that, once incorporated into daily or weekly cleaning routines, can help break the cycle of cross-contamination. The biggest misunderstanding is that many new steps and additional costs are required to properly disinfect or use protective barriers to greatly reduce the potential of cross-infection. Our society will probably never achieve pure asepsis, but in the hotel, motel, and restaurant environment we must strive to reduce the threat of potential disease transmission as much as possible. This can be accomplished by implementing a few necessary procedures and/or by using a high-level disinfectant product in a variety of ways.

SEPSIS

- Clean guest room
- Disinfect surfaces
    Toilet
    Tub/shower
    Sink and counters
    Telephone
    Floors
    Bedspread/blankets
    Pillows
    Mattress covers
- Disinfect food preparation countertops
- Disinfect food preparation utensils
- Disinfect eating utensils
- Disinfect tables or change table cloths; replace placements when applicable
- Food handling and housekeeping personnel should wear appropriate gloves
- Disinfection holding solution for silverware
- Food handling personnel pre-work scrub with antimicrobial soap
- Use antimicrobial lotion/gloves
- Follow all state codes on hygiene
- Use mattress covers and disinfect to include all bedding
- Sterilize and bag silverware where applicable

ASEPSIS

Disinfect has been substituted for the food service inspection code's *sanitize*. If proper infection-control procedures and high-level disinfection products were used by the lodging and food service industry, the number of disease outbreaks related to the hospitality industry would be greatly reduced.

Employee and Management Do's and Don'ts

DO wear hand protection when a cut, nick, or other irritation is visible.

DON'T allow exposed cuts or skin lesions the opportunity to come in contact with food or possibly touch a contaminated surface.

DO use disposable hand towels.

DON'T use cloth towels for employees or in public facilities.

DO clean and disinfect work surfaces.

DON'T use the water-only technique on work surfaces.

DO chemically treat air conditioning systems or filters.

DON'T invite stagnation in air conditioning systems.

DO follow the manufacturers' directions on contact time and temperature for effective elimination of microorganisms.

DON'T misuse disinfectant products making them ineffective.

DO practice multiple hand washing after food preparations and certain cleaning procedures.

DON'T touch faucet handles, reuse towels, or reuse soap when hand washing.

DO routinely disinfect drapes, carpets, pillows, blankets, bedspreads, and mattresses.

DON'T just vacuum carpets and allow long periods of time in between shampooing them or dry cleaning drapes,

(continued)

pillows, blankets, bedspreads, and mattresses.

DO train personnel to be aware of cross-contamination.

DON'T delegate cross-contamination procedures to untrained personnel.

DO train personnel to think about liability.

DON'T delegate anti-liability practices to untrained personnel.

DO purchase effective disinfection products.

DON'T risk liability law suits by refraining from purchasing effective disinfection products.

DO separate clean linens from soiled linens and trash on the housekeeping cart.

DON'T hang clean sheets over the waste receptacle on the housekeeping cart.

DO maintain appropriate levels of heat necessary for coffee service.

DON'T cover coffee pots with any cloth or other material to maintain heat.

DO use disinfectant presoaked table cleaning cloths to wipe smooth surface tables between customers.

DON'T wipe tables with dirty or soiled cleaning cloths.

DO use disposable disinfectant table wipes where applicable.

DON'T be negligent about wiping tables.

DO change disinfection holding solution routinely.

DON'T use past manufacturers' suggested reuse capability for disinfection holding solutions.

DO apply disinfectant to all room surfaces based on housekeeping infection-control protocol recommendations.

DON'T forget to disinfect!

DO take special care in changing the linens.

DON'T forget about the potential of infection from daily cell slough and bodily fluids on linens.

(continued)

DO apply disinfectant to telephone receiver and unit.

DON'T forget how many millions of microorganisms can be transmitted daily on the telephone receiver.

DO maintain an effective level of disinfection or sanitizing chemicals in the appropriate sink compartment.

DON'T allow negligence to cause a transmission of microorganism on improperly cleaned glasses, dishes, and silverware.

DO observe all sanitizing and disinfection principles.

DON'T be negligent about training and informing food service personnel about infection control.

DO periodic culture sample on critical surfaces or other important areas to verify chemicals' effectiveness.

DON'T use ineffective disinfection products or sanitizing chemicals.

DO purchase the least hazardous chemicals available for sanitizing and disinfecting.

DON'T create employee complaints by using toxic chemicals for sanitizing and disinfecting.

SUMMARY

1. Trained employees are a major factor in any infection-control program.
2. Personal hygiene should be constantly reinforced.
3. Proper hand washing techniques and the use of antimicrobial soap can generally eliminate 70 percent of infectious microorganisms, greatly reducing the risk of cross-infection.
4. Wall-hung or foot-activated soap/lotion dispensers and hand dryers may be cost prohibitive. A property can use other equipment, procedures, or products that are cost-effective and still break the chain of cross-infection.

REVIEW EXERCISES

1. Where applicable, employees should wear:
    a. professional uniforms
    b. street clothing
    c. disposable gowns

2. Uniforms should be:
    a. starched cotton
    b. synthetic fiber
    c. white

3. It is all right to have long hair if it is:
    a. clean and brushed
    b. covered
    c. in a bun

4. All staff should wash their hands:
    a. frequently
    b. at least three times a day
    c. never

5. Cloth towels should:
    a. not be used
    b. changed daily
    c. be used a few times

6. All soap and lotion dispensers should be:
    a. filled daily
    b. foot- or forearm-activated
    c. easily filled

5

Environmental Surface Disinfectants

KEY CONCEPTS

Surface contamination	Disinfectant
Sterilant	Precleaning
FDA (Food and Drug Administration)	EPA (Environmental Protection Agency)
OSHA (Occupational Safety and Health Administration)	CDC (Centers for Disease Control)
AOAC (Association of Official Analytical Chemists)	FIFRA (Federal Insecticide, Fungicide, Rodenticide Act (as ammended))

Many surfaces in hotels, motels, and restaurants are likely to become contaminated and should be treated by application of a chemical disinfectant to eliminate microorganisms. For example, any surface exposed to human breath, fluids, or wastes should be disinfected to protect anyone who subsequently comes in contact with it. Body fluids and wastes include blood, saliva, urine, feces, semen, and discharges from any wound or lesion.

The surfaces most frequently and heavily contaminated are those in the lavatory—the tub, commode, sink, and floor. Each can receive large doses of contaminants. The floor is also an area that can receive potential contaminants, if not properly cleaned and disinfected. The sink will receive blood and saliva during tooth brushing as well as fluids from any oral lesions such as herpes and syphillis. The commode will invariably become highly contaminated with body wastes. The tub will receive a variety of microorganisms from skin slough, discharge from lesions and wounds, occasionally some blood, and semen. Disinfection of these surfaces is absolutely necessary.

DISINFECTANTS

It is important to understand what a disinfectant is, what it can and cannot do, and how it should be used. A disinfectant is a liquid containing chemical energy that is capable of killing or inactivating certain microorganisms. It is important to differentiate between a sterilant and a disinfectant. A sterilant is capable of killing or inactivating *all* microorganisms with which it has contact—given proper use—including even the most resistant spore forms. A disinfectant can kill or inactivate some, or even most microorganisms, but not the more resistant spore forms. The effectiveness of disinfectants varies widely; some are capable of high-level disinfection, while others are relatively ineffective. The yardstick for high-level effectiveness is the ability to kill one specific pathogenic microorganism, the very resistant mycobacterium tuberculosis, or tubercle bacillus, the causative agent of tuberculosis. A disinfectant with the capability of killing both gram-negative and gram-positive bacteria is referred to as a "hospital-grade disinfectant." Virucidal and tuberculocidal activity are additional dimensions of disinfection. Most household disinfectants are capable of only low-level efficacy and leave many potentially pathogenic microorganisms untouched.

Material Safety Data Sheets (MSDS) are currently being used to comply with OSHA's Hazard Communication Standard 29 CFR 1910 1200. They identify the chemical ingredients of disinfectants and assure safe handling.

The MSDS sheets are required by OSHA to identify the hazards of all chemicals used by an employer in the workplace. The lodging and food service industry must also implement employee training and information programs to ensure that all employees are aware of the hazardous chemicals used in specific work areas. The employer must maintain a log of MSDS information received from chemical manufacturers and conduct employee training. These directives come from the Occupational Safety and Health Act of 1970 [16].

The Environmental Protection Agency is empowered to license and regulate the use of chemical disinfectants and sterilants. Any substance claiming to be either a disinfectant or a sterilant must undergo extensive testing and submit acceptable proof of testing. The specific organisms which the substance will kill or inactivate must be listed on the label as well as specific instructions regarding its preparation or mixing, use, and disposal. Use of a disinfectant for a purpose for which it is not licensed is technically a violation of Federal Law. For instance, liquids intended for disinfection of counter tops are not necessarily active enough to decontaminate medical and dental instruments. It is very important to read the label on the container to determine what level of effectiveness the product offers and how it is to be used.

PRECLEANING

The Centers for Disease Control (CDC) in Atlanta, Georgia, publishes guidelines for medical and dental facilities regarding infection-control techniques.

According to the CDC, the most important step in disinfection or sterilization is adequate precleaning of the surface or instrument. There are two reasons why precleaning is essential. If there is organic material such as blood on a surface, enormous numbers of microorganisms can be present, making effective disinfection difficult. Also, the organic material protects the microorganisms from the chemical energy of the disinfectant, again reducing the effectiveness of even the highest-level disinfectant. Thus precleaning is a necessity for maximizing the effectiveness of any disinfectant. Some disinfectants can be used for both precleaning and disinfection, because they contain a small amount of detergent. Even in this case, the disinfectant must be applied in two steps.

After the cleaning step, the disinfectant is reapplied and left wet. The chemical energy of the material is released only when the product is applied to a surface and left moist. Evaporation may take up to 30 minutes, which in a hotel or motel guest room normally is not a problem. In medical and dental situations, isopropyl alcohol is sometimes used as an environmental surface disinfectant. While it evaporates rapidly, however, allowing more efficient use of facilities, the rapid evaporation renders the alcohol nearly worthless as a disinfectant.

CHOOSING A PRODUCT

In selecting a disinfectant several criteria should be considered:

1. Is it registered with the EPA?
2. Is it tuberculocidal?
3. Is it recommended by the Centers for Disease Control?
4. Does the product application satisfy the needs of the property?
5. Is the product manufactured by a reputable company?
6. Is there documentation available from the manufacturer to verify claims?

If it satisfies these requirements, any user can be confident of its efficacy. Other factors should also be considered. The qualities of the ideal disinfectant are listed:

1. *Broad spectrum:* It kills or inactivates a broad range of microorganisms from the mycobacterium tuberculosis to most gram-negative and gram-positive bacteria.

2. *Rapid action:* It is effective in a relatively short period of time.

3. *Unaffected by contaminants:* The disinfectant should continue to be effective even in the presence of blood, saliva, feces, and so on.

4. *Nontoxic:* The product should pose no threat to either the user or anyone subsequently contacting the surface on which it is used.

5. *Nondamaging:* The product should not corrode or stain any surface on which it is used.

6. *Preparation ease:* Easy and safe to prepare (if mixing is necessary), to store, and to use.

7. *Odors:* No caustic or offensive odor.

8. *Economical:* The cost of using the product should not be prohibitively high.

9. *Long shelf life:* If there is a limited shelf life, it should be comparatively long, preferably at least a year.

LAWS AND REGULATIONS CONCERNING DISINFECTANTS

For many years, the words *disinfect* and *disinfectant* have had almost as many definitions as there are users. Since a great majority of people using disinfectants are not trained in chemistry and the medical sciences, they may be misled by interpretations that are wholly unfounded and totally untrue. It is important for people who are involved in tasks, such as decontamination of surfaces, to know both technical and legal facts. Remember that ignorance of the law is no excuse.

Definitions

Here are some legal definitions according to the U.S. Environmental Protection Agency (EPA).

Sanitize: To reduce organism count.

Disinfectant: An agent that destroys pathogenic organisms, not including spores.

Sterilant: An agent that unfailingly destroys all bacteria, mycological agents, viruses, and spores.

Federal Agencies

To understand claims and documentation associated with decontamination, one should be aware of the federal agencies that have jurisdiction in this area. The first is the U.S. Food and Drug Administration (FDA). The FDA has the authority to regulate products used in or on the body of humans or living animals. They also regulate medical devices. The Environmental Protection Agency (EPA) has the authority to regulate products used in treating the inanimate environment, including both surfaces and air. In other words, products designed for decontamination, if used in or on the living body of humans or animals, are subject to regulatory review and approval by the FDA. Products used in decontamination of the inanimate environment such as surfaces, air, objects, and so on, are subject to review, approval, and the assignment of a registration number by the EPA. The EPA registration number, once assigned, means that the producers of the product have performed all tests as defined in the Federal Insecticide, Fungicide, and Rodenticide Act (FIFRA) and the EPA guidelines. There are no other federal regulatory agencies that have jurisdiction over this type of product.

Great confusion exists concerning the role of the Centers for Disease Control. It should be noted that the CDC is not a regulatory agency and, therefore, cannot review, register, or regulate any product. The CDC can recommend the use of a product or document its effectiveness, but in order for it to do so, that product must first have been approved and registered for such use by the EPA. A great deal of confusion has arisen through the years because the CDC teaches infection control to various hospital personnel. This instructional role has sometimes included the recommendation of products used as decontaminants. This is not the legal function of the CDC, unless the products have already met federal standards administered by the EPA and are duly registered for the use stated on the product label.

The only regulatory authority covering disinfectants recommended for treating inanimate environmental surfaces is the EPA. The Association of Official Analytical Chemists (AOAC) is the only recognized organization that establishes the testing standards followed by the EPA. If tests are performed by independent laboratories or other groups of researchers that do not follow AOAC guidelines, the claims are not considered valid. The AOAC is responsible for defining which tests are acceptable; the EPA is responsible for monitoring and approving valid test results based on the AOAC standards.

We constantly see instances in the commercial market, as well as in government, of nonapproved labeling and product misuse. The legal definition of *disinfectant* is given above. A *general disinfectant* is further defined as one that has passed the AOAC Use-Dilution Test for *Staphylococcus aureus* and *Salmonella cholereasuis*, has been subjected to several pharmacological tests to determine its potential toxic effects on humans, and is registered with the EPA. The official definition of a *hospital or medical disinfectant* is one that has successfully passed the AOAC Use-Dilution Test covering *Staphylococcus aureus*, *Salmonella cholereasuis*, *Pseudomonas aeruginosa*, and the *Mycobacterium tuberculosis*, has also been subjected to toxicity testing, and is registered with the EPA as a high-grade disinfectant.

Misleading Labels and Unsupported Claims

To merely state on the label of the container that a product is a disinfectant, without making available the efficacy and toxicity data which determine effectiveness and safety of use, is illegal. Some companies may pass certain AOAC tests allowing for certain claims against specific bacteria or viruses; bleach, for example, makes claims against Staphylococcus, influenza A2, Hong Kong, Rhinovirus 17, Streptococcus, and foot fungus. Based on the test, the EPA approves bleach for certain household disinfectant capabilities. However, according to the label, no claim was made against Herpes I and II or other viruses or the TB mycobacterium. If this product is used and a transmission problem occurs, the manufacturer is not liable, because any use of the product not recommended on the label is a misuse of the product. The organisms against which the product was tested may or may not be specified on the label after approval by the EPA. If the option to claim efficacy against particular organisms is chosen, only the organisms tested may be listed on the label.

The EPA guidelines together with the FIFRA, constitute the

law for these products and law applies to everyone without exception. Numerous articles have been published stating that the decontamination of manikins used by the Red Cross for CPR training can be accomplished with either alcohol or chlorine. Neither alcohol nor chlorine are cleaners and we have seen no appropriate test data suggesting that either can be safely and effectively used for this purpose. Yet, both products have been used without proper documentation for approximately 90 years.

Other products may also test and receive EPA approval and then omit certain information from the product label or container. A product may be tuberculocidal and have passed a test when heated to 77°F, but may represent the TB claim without specifically stating the need for heat and additional exposure time for total elimination of the bacteria.

In response to widespread misapprehensions of this kind, an article in the *Federal Register* dated October 24, 1984 defined this entire picture. The article, entitled *Environmental Protection Agency*, Part II 40 CFR Part 158 data requirements for pesticide registration, refers to the *Pesticide Assessment Guidelines*, subdivision G, product performance, U.S. EPA, Washington, D.C., November 1982. The pesticide guidelines include procedures for testing all disinfectants, and clearly prescribe the requirement for establishing effectiveness and safety of use. This document covers methods of developing efficacy data, culture media, and ATCC culture numbers, as well as very specific functional testing requirements which must be met before applying for EPA approval. Page 16 of the article clearly defines the disinfectant definitions noted earlier in this chapter.

Research in decontamination and disinfection, like all research, must follow uniform guidelines or it has little or no practical value. Studies not following EPA protocol have been conducted in academic institutions from time to time and the results and recommendations have been published. Occasionally, the practices they recommend are actually applied in their institutions. Even some epidemiologists have published recommendations without any documentation. These cannot be considered reliable or responsible statements.

CAVEAT EMPTOR—BUYER, BEWARE!

Anyone performing decontamination with disinfectants should first check the product label for an EPA registration number. They should then read the label to determine what the product covers. In other words, if a label claims effectiveness against *Staphylococcus aureus* or *Salmonella cholereasuis*, one cannot assume that any other organisms are effected. If an organism is not clearly listed on the label and the user is not familiar with EPA test requirements for hospital and general disinfectants, he cannot take for granted that the product will destroy that organism. Information should be sought by calling the EPA directly. As a microbiologist once said, "If it isn't on the label, it hasn't been tested."

Chlorine has often been considered effective against hepatitis, TB, Salmonella, Staphylococcus, and Streptococcus. Even the largest producers of chlorine do not make total kill claims on the labels of their containers. The chlorine manufacturers say nothing beyond *disinfectant* or *sanitize* depending upon the recommended dilution on their labels. Some companies with private labels or who provide generic products, do not even have an EPA registration identification number on the label nor do they make any specific viral or bacteriological claims. Using chlorine or sodium hypochlorite products is not contraindicated as a means for disinfecting environmental surfaces; just be sure the product is used according to its labeling and EPA registration number. The use of a product in an inconsistent manner to the labeling is in violation of Federal Law. Again, the manufacturer is not held liable, only the people or property misusing the product. This is why OSHA now requires all employees to have hazard communication training regarding hazardous chemicals used in the workplace. Do not be caught unaware; over 2,000 chemicals and substances are considered hazardous. Chemicals like janitorial supplies, correction fluids, pool additives, pesticides, drain cleaners/degreasers, surface disinfectants, and many more are on the OSHA list.

The general public, and particularly the hospitality industry, must be able to recognize unreliable labeling and undocumented recommendations in the literature. Unsubstantiated claims for chlorine as a disinfectant create a false sense of security for the users and can lead to serious repercussions. Beware of statements like "We haven't heard of any problems, whatever they are." The lodging and hospitality industry has already experienced and documented problems with such viral and bacteriological diseases as Legionnaires, Hepatitis A, and Salmonella poisoning. The media coverage of AIDS has created a new fear of contamination in consumers, employers, and employees. The time to address proper infection-control procedures and establish a better defense against liability is *now!*

Housekeeping and food and beverage areas and personnel are at a moderate risk level daily. Property owners have a responsibility to both their employees and their guests to be proactive and not reactive about potential cross-infection.

As an industry, we should take the initiative before OSHA or another agency begins to regulate our businesses. As we saw in Chapter 2, recurrent infections in the medical and dental care fields have motivated OSHA to become more involved in monitoring procedures and the proper use of disinfection products. The similarities of lodging and hospitality industry facilities to those of hospitals, nursing homes, and other health-related institutions invite government involvement.

In contacting the CDC and asking specifically what guidelines exist for hotels, motels, and restaurants regarding infection-control procedures, it was not reassuring to find out that no specific guidelines exist. The CDC said that guidelines for effective procedures are controlled by the FDA. In contacting the FDA, a proposed Food Protection Unicode was obtained and reviewed for guidelines. The basics are covered in a one-page chapter on employee health, personal cleanliness, and hygiene practices. In further review of the code, the FDA defined sanitation as the act of reducing microbial organisms on cleaned food-contact surfaces to a safe level, requiring a test demonstrating a reduction in either *Escherichia coli* or *Staphylococcus aureus* within 30 seconds. Salmonella was not mentioned as being tested.

In Chapter 5 of the proposed Food Protection Unicode, chlorine solutions specifically are required to have a minimum of 10 seconds contact time, provide a specific pH, specific water temperature, and a specific concentration (parts per million [ppm]) of free chlorine to be used. In observing many two- and three-component sink operations, rarely are all of the highly technical, very specific time, pH, and water temperature considerations closely followed. Remember these are only sanitation guidelines which, as defined by the FDA, is the act of reducing microbial organisms on cleaned food contact surfaces to a safe level. Can the same "safe" level be achieved in a sink compartment?

Consider that the model sanitation code developed by the Public Health Services goes back over 60 years to the early 1920s. The Public Health Services' codes relating to food protection and sanitation in food service establishments were initiated in 1934. Revisions and expansion of these codes have occurred since 1938. In 1968, the FDA assumed the responsibility of the retail food protection program and updated the food service sanitation code in 1976. The new unicode is based on the efforts of a task force assembled from industry, government, and third party regulatory officials. The new unicode addresses the same issues of time and temperature, food han-

dling, preparation, storage, and so on. Guidelines and procedures are just like computer programs: only as good as the
people implementing the tasks or following directions. Since
effective sanitation relies on people to follow directions, it is
the people who need to become more aware of why infection-
control procedures and the use of high-level disinfection
products will help reduce the risk of disease transmission. The
people in the food service industry must be educated and then
motivated about proper procedures, because it is people that
continue to cause the majority of the problems relating to
food-borne illnesses.

DISINFECTANT REVIEW

Disinfection is a process in which some, or even most, microorganisms are destroyed, but not the most resistant spore forming
organisms.

Disinfectants are liquids or aerosol sprays which contain
chemical energy capable of killing or irreversibly inactivating
certain organisms.

1. Disinfectants used by business and industry should be
   high-level and capable of killing the mycobacterium tuberculosis at use-dilution and should be so indicated on the
   label. Recently, the EPA approved over 40 companies that
   tested and killed the AIDS virus on a surface. The CDC felt
   if a product was capable of killing TB, it would also kill
   AIDS. The AIDS virus is easier to kill on a surface than TB,
   but should not be the primary concern of a high-level
   disinfectant.

2. Disinfectants should all be registered with the EPA and dis-
   play the EPA registration number on the label or container.

3. Chemical disinfectants are licensed for use in a specific

application and must not be used for any purpose nor in any manner not recommended by the manufacturer.

Disinfection Product Applications

1. All environmental surfaces
2. Holding or immersion solutions prior to warewashing (food service)
3. Laundry additives (food service and lodging)
4. Health care applications

INFECTION-CONTROL PRODUCT UPDATE: TECHNOLOGY BREAKTHROUGH

The twenty-first century is nearly upon us, promising new challenges, technologies, and opportunities. The EPA, OSHA, and the FDA are all regulatory agencies concerned with our health, safety, and environment. Our food, medication, and air quality are the focus of much research.

Our society has focused on reducing our cholesterol intake, exercising, avoiding the use of drugs, minimizing the risk of disease transmission, and not smoking cigarettes. More research is being conducted on dealing with hazardous waste and reusing garbage for creating new sources of energy. Ongoing projects concerning the ozone layer of our atmosphere continue to target the use of freon and aerosol products as the main reasons for its reduction.

Currently, various companies doing extensive research

on ionization systems. Electrical ionization or altering charges of air-borne particles (including dust, pollen, smoke, elemental metals, virus, sporogenic organisms, and other particulates) has been promoted as a very effective method for controlling contamination.

This specific technology has applications in all aspects of health care, manufacturing, hospitality businesses, and even offers applications for athletic training and use in school gyms. Particles are actually collected on special positive grid collectors, where they are rendered electrically inert. There are no motors, fans, filters, air movement, noise, moving parts, electrode erosion, particle precipitation, nor electrical "spiking." It is simply a system designed to enhance air quality and to create the optimum environment.

Think of the benefits, in food processing plants and smoking areas in hotels, motels, and restaurants or in your home or car, of eliminating contaminants and possibly reducing allergic reactions and exposure to disease causing microorganisms.

This innovative ionization process may be a major breakthrough for twentieth century technology. It is worthy of our honorable mention toward better infection-control techniques available for all business and industry.

By integrating a *clean room* concept in future buildings, factories, and public facilities, our society would be making great strides toward solving some of our environmental problems such as smog, acid rain, and disease transmission, and the high cost of health care. The EPA has indicated that indoor air quality pollution levels can exceed the standard of outdoor air up to 100 times. The hazards faced by all who breathe, are considerable. If you are concerned about your health or the safety and health of your employees, contact the J.D. Group, Inc. to request information on a specific system that is applicable for your business or home.

High-level disinfection infection-control products, with food service and housekeeping applications and employee training programs, are available from the following companies:

- The J.D. Group, Infection Control Training Specialists, in-house training for housekeepers, food service workers, and nursing home staffs: Seminars for business and industry—certified and endorsed by the American Dieticians Association, National Executive Housekeepers Association, National Environmental Health Association, and Institute of Applied Studies (2101 Eastern Boulevard, York, Pennsylvania 17402 [717-755-7512] or 162 Newton Street, Brooklyn, New York 11122 [718-388-9435]).

- Ray Industries, Disinfectant Chemicals, Waterless Antiseptic Hand Cleaner (1558 Bonnie Road, Macedonia, Ohio 44056).

- K-Zyme Laboratories, Drain Cleaner, Degreasers, Antimicrobial Soap (P.O. Box 802, Salem, Virginia 24153).

Infection-control seminars are offered through many colleges and universities that have hotel and restaurant management programs. Contact the continuing education department, the hotel and restaurant department, or travel and tourism department of a school in your vicinity and find out when infection-control educational programs will be offered. The programs offer certification for members of the American Dieticians Association, National Executive Housekeepers Association, and National Environmental Health Association.

Categories of Disinfection Solutions

Advantages

Glutaraldehydes formulations: primarily for medical and dental instruments; does not tarnish most metals

Alcohols: easy to use; fairly drying to hands and skin

Hydrogen peroxide: very stable

Phenols: fairly stable; depends upon the formulation; some phenolics are effective against virus and most bacteria; other phenolics remain at only household strength disinfectants

Formaldehyde: none

Iodophors: economical; bio-cidal activity occurs within approximately 30 minutes; easily mixed with water

Disadvantages

Relatively expensive; can sensitize skin on repeated contact; vapors may irritate eyes and nose

Limited antimicrobial spectrum; dries very rapidly; flammable

Rapidly inactivated by catalase and still under-going research as a sterilant

Studies indicate that phenols are irregularly virucidal, potentially irritating to the skin, and damaging to certain metals; phenols may cause irritation in older persons resulting in respiratory problems

Flammable colorless gas having a strong pungent, suffocating odor; extremely irritating to the skin

Solutions somewhat unstable; solutions may temporarily stain; contact time and dilution must be strictly followed

(continued)

Advantages	**Disadvantages**
Chlorine compounds: fast action broad-spectrum biocides	Persistent odor; can corrode metals; irritates skin and eyes
Sodium hypochlorite (household bleach): when used in conjunction with a thorough cleansing procedure, it disinfects surfaces in 3 to 30 minutes, depending on the amount of debris and virus present	Highly corrosive to some metals; solution tends to be unstable; may eventually cause cracks in plastics; caustic to skin and eyes; strong unpleasant odor
Chlorine dioxide: can be used to disinfect nonmetal items; mixed with water; does not discolor skin	Freshly prepared solution required for each process; biocidal activity of solution may decline after more than 14 days of storage
Acid chlorite: Good anti-microbial activity	Requires very careful dilution; in solutions stored for more than one day, its activity diminishes and develops an increasingly strong chlorine odor

QUATERNARY AMMONIUM COMPOUNDS: "SUPER QUATS"

The older quat compounds without synergistic fortified additives were considered to have a very low biocidal activity, and solutions could support the growth of gram-negative bacteria. Some of these basic quaternary compounds are still being used and causing problems, but a new generation of quat chemicals that meet CDC guidelines for high-level disinfectants are emerging.

These new Super Quats have combined the basic gentle and pleasant advantages with better killing chemicals to provide the best of both worlds: easy to use and effective against TB; they combine excellent cleaning capabilities with high-level disinfection, are ready-to-use, and in some cases diluted one to one with applications from floor mopping to surface disinfecting.

SUMMARY

1. Surface disinfection is highly desirable in public facilities.
2. The EPA controls the licensing and use of disinfectants.
3. Precleaning of surfaces before disinfection is essential.
4. The properties of the ideal disinfectant are as follows:
   - broad range of microorganisms killed
   - works rapidly
   - tolerates contaminants such as blood and soap
   - nontoxic
   - nondamaging
   - easy and safe to prepare, store, and use
   - inoffensive odor
   - economical
   - long shelf life
5. There are clear federal guidelines for testing and documenting the effectiveness of disinfectant products.
6. Chlorine and alcohol, although popularly believed to be disinfectants, are not registered with the EPA for total effi-

cacy against all viral and bacteriological microorganisms that cause infections.

7. If the hospitality industry does not take a proactive stance regarding disinfection, OSHA can be expected to intervene as it has in the dental and health care industries.

8. The selection and use of specific high-level disinfection chemicals depends a great deal on the type of operation involved. Housekeeping products for various applications will be covered in Chapter 6 and food service applications in Chapter 7. In general, the selection of products should conform to some of the guidelines defined in Chapter 5. What to look for: follow the manufacturers' directions for required contact time and read the label. You may have to educate your distributor's sales representative as to what you need and why, but you will at least have his or her attention based on your new knowledge of infection control and high-level disinfection products.

REVIEW EXERCISES

1. Why is disinfection of surfaces in public facilities highly desirable?

2. What is a disinfectant?

3. What is the test to determine if a disinfectant is a "hospital grade" material?

4. Why is it important to read the label on the disinfectant container?

5. Why is precleaning essential prior to surface disinfection?

6. Why must a disinfectant be left wet on the surface being treated?

7. What are the main points which should be considered in determining the acceptability of a disinfectant?

6

Guest Room Disinfection

KEY CONCEPTS

Clean	Sanitize	Barriers
Bacteriostat	Disinfect	Liability

The knowledge of infectious diseases is abundant and how to control or reduce infectious disease is a serious concern. In the lodging industry, there are four species of housekeeping managers. The "I can't afford it" species, the "I'll offend my customers" species, the "I don't know how to" species, and the "nothing has happened to me" species. The "bury your head in the sand" or "ostrich syndrome" needs further examination. Most properties feel comfortable that they are cleaning and sanitizing and not exposed to any risk from disease transmission. After we examine the "ostrich syndrome" more closely, this chapter will heighten your awareness about the disease transmission risk factors that occur daily for the housekeeper and/or the guest. First we discuss how steps can be taken to eliminate the "ostrich syndrome" to provide proper infection control for the employees and customers of lodging establishments.

The "I can't afford it" species clearly illustrates the possibility of a liability suit. Comparing law suits to the cost of disinfection products, which in most cases replace products currently purchased for housekeeping functions, is no contest. Tally the actual cost of current supplies as compared to effective disinfection products and a quick extinction of the "I can't afford it" syndrome will occur.

The "I'll offend my customers" species probably is not aware that the customer is already concerned and confused about disease transmission and is looking for answers. Infection-control procedures and the use of high-level disinfection products will not offend anyone, but should show that the property is concerned and doing everything to offer accommodations worthy of a return visit. When infection control is properly introduced, the overall gain is one of appreciation, respect, and support from both the employee and guests.

The "I don't know how" species, is really asking for direction. These housekeepers or decision makers should attend an infection-control seminar or read this manual. Once they understand the purpose of infection control procedures and the need for high-level disinfection as a part of routine housekeeping functions, this species disappears forever.

The "nothing can happen to me" species request a special tact. Fortunately, the room side of the industry is far less documented to have caused major problems of disease outbreaks, the worst scenario being the Legionnaires' Convention in Philadelphia, which led to the identification of a new bacteria and the deaths of convention attendees. Other minor incidences of scabies or water-transmitted infections have been linked to lodging establishments, but nothing drastic enough to force change. The industry must be educated and made aware of the potential threats that exist from disease transmission. There are still properties being closed when linked to new bacteria or viruses. Legionnaires has not been controlled and two-thirds of the hotel properties utilize an evaporative cooling tower system for air conditioning. Based on the amount of liability insurance paid yearly by major property corporations, if a chance to reduce these premiums existed because of a change in employee training or the use of better more-efficient products, this species would be better protected from the possibilities of being the first hotel or motel linked to a major hepatitis, AIDS, or another Legionnaires outbreak. The consumer species is more aware of problems and looking for a reason to stay in the same facility repeatedly if a comfort level has been established due to efforts by the property to reduce the risk of disease transmission.

The guest room in a hotel or motel may be the last place one would expect to find potential infectious diseases because rooms are cleaned daily. However, let's examine the normal room cleaning ritual, the 10 to 20 minute routine performed by the housekeeper. Each property may have in place a set of guidelines or particular step-by-step cleaning procedures. In most cases, the following occurs in all rooms:

1. The room is vacuumed.
2. The sheets and pillow cases are changed.
3. All surfaces are dusted.
4. All towels and amenities are replaced.
5. The tub and shower are cleaned and rinsed.
6. The toilet and sinks are wiped and cleaned.
7. Mirrors are cleaned.
8. Trash is removed.
9. A final inspection is made by the supervisor.

Now the room is ready for a new occupant. The next guest may be a disease carrier, because 20 percent of the population harbors some type of infectious disease [17].

This makes the room a potential breeding ground for microbial pathogens.

This can be attributed to the fact that usually the cleaning supplies used in guest rooms are household or industrial-grade cleaning supplies. These materials may, in fact, kill some bacteria, like Salmonella or Pseudomonas, but they have not been tested by the EPA for high-level disinfection capability. To pass the EPA test for household-level disinfectants a product must kill two of the three main strains of bacteria: *Pseudomonas aeruginosa, Salmonella cholereasuis,* and *Staphylococcus aureus.*

These bacteria can promote infections, but are not difficult to kill. The EPA requirements for high-level (hospital grade) disinfectants are much more stringent. They require elimination of all microorganisms up to and including the *Mycobacterium tuberculosis.* This is considered the most difficult bacterium to kill without complete sterilization.

Let's examine what was *not* done by the housekeeper:

1. No appropriate disinfectants were used on any surfaces.
2. The bedspread or blanket was not treated or cleaned.
3. The mattress cover, if present, was not treated.
4. The telephone was not sprayed with a disinfectant.
5. All of the cleaned bathroom areas were rinsed with water, which carries new bacteria. In some areas even the treated water used in homes and businesses contains contaminants, and these bacteria could potentially recontaminate a clean surface.
6. Even though the carpets were vacuumed, no disinfection steps were taken.
7. The housekeeper probably did not use gloves or other hand protection to provide a barrier against cross-infection. If a nick, cut, rash, or skin problem exists, gloves should be mandatory for the housekeeper's protection.

Further, while the guest room in our example may have been cleaned by a product generating lots of suds, it can still harbor pathogens looking for a host. Currently, most cleaning products are diluted from a concentrate; this preparation process diminishes their capability of inactivating or destroying pathogenic microorganisms.

IMPROVING GUEST ROOM DISINFECTION

One of the goals of an infection-control program is breaking the cycle of infection and eliminating cross-contamination by reducing the number of pathogenic organisms. This can be done by incorporating proper disinfection procedures into the housekeeping regime, in addition to providing barriers to infection for both the staff and guests. One such barrier benefiting the guests would be an additional sheet on top of the blankets creating a sandwich effect. Bedspreads and blankets are prime collectors of sloughed cells, possibly containing pathogenic organisms. Also, sometimes sexual acts occur on top of bedspreads and blankets which results in body fluids contaminating them. Since blankets and bedspreads are not changed daily as are bed linens, the addition of a second sheet, changed daily, is a desirable and necessary safeguard for the protection of the guests.

In most cases, a combination disinfectant/detergent should replace current cleaning products. The industrial-strength cleaners now used in most hotels, motels, and restaurants have been tested in most cases for their ability to kill Salmonella, Staphylococcus, or Streptococcus. There is also the possibility of incorporating one or two available products in addition to current cleaning supplies. Either way, the more effective products should be incorporated into the daily routine. Without them, cleaning is only the removal of dirt, not the removal of infectious disease-causing organisms.

You may ask why we need proper disinfection. Consider that the average adult mouth contains 160 septillion (160,000,000,000,000,000,000,000,000) microorganisms [18].* These organisms may include those that cause hepatitis, syphillis, or tuberculosis. Surfaces may harbor fewer organisms than the human body, but the potential for cross-infection still

*Reprinted with permission from *The Journal of Dental Research* (42) 509–520, 1963.

exists, because people are on the go from place to place, and all microorganisms that hitch-hike end up on a surface. In a housekeeping or food and beverage area, the employee as well as the guest is a vulnerable target for pathogenic organisms.

Diseases Potentially Transmitted in a Room Environment

Cold
Flu
Tuberculosis
Herpes
Staphylococcus Infections
Streptococcus Infections
Hepatitis
AIDS
Athlete's Foot
Legionnaires' Disease

Risk Situations in Which Disease Can Be Transmitted in a Housekeeping Function to an Employee

A. Moist towels
B. Body fluids on environmental surfaces, toilet seats, sink, sheets, tub, shower
C. Bed wetter
D. Vomit
E. Soap soup
F. Air conditioning systems
G. Accumulation of airborne organisms on surfaces, drapes, bedspreads

---

Risk to Guest from Room Occupancy

A. Sink
B. Toilet
C. Telephone
D. Mattress
E. Air Conditioner
F. Tub/shower
G. Carpet
H. Drinking glasses
I. Towels, washcloths, laundry

A Scenario

Upon arriving in a New York City hotel room, after extensive tipping, the bellman opens your room door and you find some left-behind debris. Did the housekeeper forget it? Probably not. Chances are that the previous guest re-entered the room after checking out and, before a final room check, you checked in. Who was there before you? What precautions does the hotel take in its housekeeping procedures? Is it true that some house-keepers don't even have a cleaning solution on the cart and just rinse sinks and tubs, dust, change linens, vacuum, and go on to the next room? This is certainly not standard procedure, but, in reality, it occurs more often than it should.

Beyond "Clean"

The appearance of a guest room is vital to a property's image. Since more and more consumers are becoming cautious about disease transmission and research is unable to answer all the questions, the time has come to be concerned about what lies beneath the surface impressions of style, charm, and tidiness. AIDS, hepatitis, Legionnaires, Herpes, Salmonella poisoning, and Pseudomonas infections have become a part of daily realities. The microorganisms that surround us in our environment must not be ignored, nor should we become paranoid. We simply need to act, not react, to prevent possible infections. We have the capability to reduce the risk of infection and eliminate the growth of microorganisms. Housekeeping on a daily basis assures cleanliness. Why not take clean to the next level of protection for the guests and staff members?

In the average room of a hotel, motel, inn, or resort property, we find the same basic furnishing—bed, dresser, table, chairs, telephone, television, desk, closet, bathroom, fixtures, rugs, drapes, heater/air conditioner, and lamps. The quality and style of the furnishings may vary, but the same pieces exist. Let's examine how these furnishings provide a mode of transmission for bacterial and viral diseases. The human body is the main mode of transmission for viral and bacteriological disease, for the body constantly sheds old and dead cells as well as hair. Remember that all organisms are hitchhikers with no means of propulsion. Therefore, they ride on particulate matter in air, moisture, particles, or dust. Eventually, these particles settle on surfaces. The surfaces in a room environment—the rug, furniture, exposed floors, bathroom sink, tub, toilet, towels, telephone, drapes, bedspread, blankets, mattress, dresser or desk, lamps, and, last but not least, the door knob—are all potential cracks and corners for disease-harboring organisms. Do you want to stay in a room that has only been "cleaned?"

Clean: to remove visible dirt and debris

Bacteriostat: stops organisms from reproducing; does not kill, simply inhibits growth

Sanitize: to reduce the number of organisms to safe levels

(continued)

Disinfect: to kill all organisms, except spores, which require sterilization to deactivate or eliminate. The three grades of disinfectant are:

a. High-level, hospital-grade: must kill three organisms—*Staphylococcus aureus, Salmonella cholerasuis, Pseudomonas aeruginosa*—plus these organisms: tuberculosis, pathogenic fungus, and viruses.
b. General household disinfectant: must kill two organisms, Staphylococcus and Salmonella.
c. Limited disinfectant: must kill only Salmonella.

The following chart, part of a culture series taken at a major hotel, reflects the presence of many organisms too numerous to count (TNTC). After application of a disinfectant or protective barrier like the Phone-Shield™ on the public phone, the organism count was greatly reduced and, in most cases, eliminated.

HOUSEKEEPING SURFACES TESTED

Place of Sampling	(Before) Control Plate Count/Organism Identified	(After) Test Plate Count/Organism Identified
House phone (lobby)	TNTC*/Gram-positive Staphylococcus	2/Gram-positive rods
Pay phone	57/Gram-positive Staphylococcus	0
Toilet seat (hotel room)	TNTC/Gram-positive Staphylococcus	0
Public toilet seat	TNTC/Gram-positive Staphylococcus	0
Urinal handle (public)	TNTC/Gram-negative rods, Gram-positive Diplococci	0
Light switch	TNTC/Gram-positive rods	0

*TNTC—too numerous to count.

Disinfection is a necessary step to complete the cleaning process. We provide a case in point. Two housekeepers enter a hotel room. One is responsible for the bathroom and the other for the bed and living area. The bathroom housekeeper removes a clean, unused towel and wipes all surfaces in the tub/shower, removes the soap, wipes off the sink and counter, and replaces all towels. Not one type of cleaning product is utilized. Is this a time-saving exercise? The second housekeeper removes the bed sheets and pillow cases, takes the cleaning cloth from her waist, wipes off the headboards and end tables, straightens the litera-ture on the desk, and proceeds to make the bed. Since it is a king-size bed, she crawls across it to straighten the clean sheets. These procedures are not recommended, but they still take place. This is why disinfection of some type is necessary in order to eliminate liability due to human error.

Avoiding Risk

The housekeeper should be aware of the personal risk involved on a daily basis. If any exposed nicks, cuts, skin irritation, or open wounds are present or occur during daily cleaning proce-dures, the housekeeper should wear latex gloves or some type of hand protection to eliminate the potential of cross-infection.

In the medical profession, three cases of AIDS transmission have been reported to the Centers for Disease Control in which just the blood of an AIDS victim was splattered on the skin of nurses. Within a relatively short period of time all of the nurses tested positive [19].

In a housekeeping parallel, how often is blood present from shaving nicks on surfaces or on used moist bath towels? How often is contact made by the unsuspecting housekeeper? Proper disinfection and barrier protection greatly reduces the risk of transmission.

Introducing Disinfectant Products

The application of high-level hospital-grade disinfectant products either with or in place of current cleaning supplies requires no special skill or training. The routine is the same; the disinfectants protect the innocent. If proper disinfection procedures have been established and the most effective product available is integrated into the daily room routine, only a positive result occurs. With the right product, even an every-other-day routine provides better protection than soap and water or other household disinfectants. Some housekeepers use ammonia or bleach in a diluted form and feel comfortable. They also have a constant companion because the odor of bleach or ammonia stays with them. Even though these chemicals, when diluted, may have a limited capability of removing or inhibiting bacteria, the toxic and corrosive effects on users and surfaces are not a positive marketing tool. In a recent employee training seminar, housekeepers expressed concerns about chemical odors and the toxicity of currently used cleaning supplies, mentioning that they were constantly getting headaches. It was recommended to the property that less-toxic chemicals should be found in order to reduce the possibility of employee complaints to OSHA.

The following procedures show effective application of disinfectant products. If a property decides to use only high-level disinfection chemicals in adjunct with current cleaning supplies, the application is easy. After precleaning the bathroom, a light application of the disinfectant on all surfaces is all that is required. The product should be sprayed or wiped on and left to air dry. This application provides a protective barrier from any contamination. In the room itself, the disinfectant should be used on drapes, air conditioners, telephones, rugs, blankets, mattress or mattress covers, and bedspreads. Multipurpose disinfectants can be used in most spray applications for rug and furniture cleaning. Even if an additive is used in the evaporative air conditioning system, a disinfectant may be applied to individual room units on a routine basis. The proper application of a high-level disinfectant provides a means of reducing the microorganism population.

AVOIDING LIABILITY AND ADVERSE PUBLICITY

Person to person, person to surface, surface to person, and person to object all are modes of transmission that exist on a daily basis. Why not protect your employees and guests on a daily basis? If your property establishes an infection-control program and uses high-level disinfectant products, it will be more difficult for a liability suit against the property to succeed. Proof beyond a shadow of a doubt will have to be used as hard evidence in a transmission case. Remember, once a property, or the entire lodging and hospitality industry, establishes a standard of excellence, any lawsuit must prove negligence. Your infection-control protocol shows your concern for the welfare of the customer. Only properties not regularly using an effective infection-control program and products will be subject to lawsuits.

OSHA has been given expanded authority to investigate and monitor working conditions that deal with a predictable risk for disease transmission. These areas include housekeeping and laundry operations. The transmission of viral and bacteriological organisms that results in illness or infections are being closely scrutinized and are receiving media attention, as a result of the world AIDS problem. The modes of transmission of AIDS are not thoroughly understood. It primarily is thought to be transmitted by sexual activity or other percutaneous avenues relating to drug use or blood transfusion. The disease is obviously carried in blood and semen but has been found to exist in other body fluids, as well. For housekeepers or laundry workers, the potential to come into contact with bodily fluids or infectious organisms on surfaces definitely exists. Caution and an established infection-control regime are the best course of protection.

How often are the blankets, bedspreads, pillows, and drapes cleaned? What is being done to reduce the microbial life that lands on these surfaces daily from human cell slough, sneezing, coughing, perspiring, and so on? Who is the judge and jury on infection-control techniques? Are we going to continue to ask ourselves the same questions? Are we going to take for granted that "nothing will happen to me?" The time to address infection is now, not when someone sues the property for food poisoning, disease transmission, or worse.

High Stakes, Simple Precautions

Hotel industry revenues are $45 billion annually and growing. Every year, more rooms are added requiring more housekeeping, laundry, food preparation, and other daily activities which continue to contribute to potential cross-contamination from guests and employees. Until all the questions can be answered about viral and bacteriological organisms and related diseases, a need exists for creating a standard for infection control.

The application of the appropriate disinfectants is simply a matter of *doing:* act versus react; take a stand on improving clean surfaces; improve sanitation. Properly disinfected surfaces provide your employees and guests with a healthy environment. Bring your guests back by providing them with a reason to believe in your concern. Discounts, free trips, and other promotional gimmicks are effective, but good health and proper hygiene ensure a safer environment, which allows for a personal comfort level guaranteed to generate customer satisfaction. The housekeeping staff also can look forward to a healthier, safer working atmosphere, fewer sick days, and better employee–employer relations. A reliable disinfection program plays an important role in presenting the property's image of hospitality.

Product Application—Housekeeping

1. Types of disinfectants
    A. Spray-aerosol/non-aerosol pump
    B. Liquid multipurpose (bulk)
    C. Disposable wipes
    D. Antimicrobial cleaning lotion
    E. Drain cleaner/sanitizer concentrate
2. Applications
    A. All surfaces (bathroom, dressers, telephone, and so on): daily or routinely depending upon infection control protocol
    B. Blankets, spread, mattress covers
    C. Air conditioner, filters (spray); evaporative cooling systems (additive)
    D. Carpets, drapes
    E. Employee hand washing protection
3. Certain high-level hospital disinfectants are multipurpose. They can replace glass cleaners and furniture polish, fight odors, reduce or eliminate mold, mildew, and fungus, or can be used in combination with other cleaning supplies.

Application Instructions for Multipurpose Disinfectants

1. When multipurpose disinfectants are being used only as the final step in the cleaning process, apply only a light spray, for 3 to 4 seconds on the surface; allow to air dry.

2. When a multipurpose disinfectant is used as a glass cleaner or furniture polish, use normal cleaning procedures, apply to the surface, and wipe off.

3. When a multipurpose disinfectant is used to remove mold and mildew, use "elbow-grease" depending on the severity of the build-up; when routinely used these products eliminate growth of the fungus.

4. When a multipurpose disinfectant is used to eliminate odors, apply three to four light sprays into the air over the bed, in the bathroom, and in the closet and door entry areas.

Infection-Control Protocol: General Recommendations for Lodging Establishments

Amenities—for disinfection and personal protection
Barrier protection for employees
Antimicrobial soaps
Use of high-level disinfection products
Proper OSHA compliance training program for
        employees
Ongoing training programs
Proper hand washing techniques
Routine Legionnaires' test and chemical applications

SUMMARY

1. Housekeepers are exposed to infection on a daily basis. Hand protection should be required and properly explained. Your employees' safety is always an issue.
2. The cleaning products in current use may kill some bacteria but not the more resistant microorganisms.
3. High-level disinfectant products can easily be incorporated into the daily cleaning routine.
4. It is necessary to routinely disinfect mattresses, drapes, rugs, blankets, bedspreads, pillows, and other surfaces that are not changed daily in a room.
5. Bedspreads, blankets, and mattresses are high-risk items for the potential transmission of infection because they are not laundered daily, as are sheets, leaving millions of cells sloughed by each room occupant.

REVIEW EXERCISES

1. Twenty percent of the entire population carries some type of infectious disease:

   True or False?

2. A clean surface is a disinfected surface:

   True or False?

3. Bedspreads are cleaned daily:

   True or False?

4. Industrial-strength cleaning supplies have been EPA tested for effectiveness against:
   a. AIDS
   b. hepatitis

    c. Salmonella

5. A hotel or motel room is free from potential infectious organisms:

True or False?

6. A housekeeper with a cut or nick on the hand should:

    a. wear hand protection
    b. use antimicrobial soap
    c. use a hand lotion
    d. all of the above

7. A high-grade disinfectant meets EPA test requirements against:

    a. *Mycobacterium tuberculosis*
    b. hepatitis
    c. the common cold

7

Food and Beverage Areas

KEY CONCEPTS

Surface Disinfection	Barrier Protection
Presoaking	

The hotel food and beverage director and the restaurateur have the most reason for concern about proper infection control. Every day employees and guests are constantly moving in and out of critical areas. Food handlers are preparing vegetables and fruits; the tables are constantly being reset to accommodate new customers. Dishes and silverware are being dropped; the kitchen personnel are hot and perspiring; the waiters and waitresses are hurriedly covering their stations, trying to serve guests with quick service and a smile. The attention given to detail regarding personal hygiene, proper sanitation, or infec-tion-control procedures is far less than the attention paid to the customer by a server trying to establish a rapport and provide good service to generate a gratuity. Hospitality is the key, and food and beverage generates the revenues.

Hotels offer many kinds of services, such as gourmet restaurants and sports facilities, to attract business. Studies have shown that business travelers stay at different locations when they return to the same destination. Much of the burden in this constant battle for customer loyalty falls heavily on food and beverage. The other constant battle involves dealing with humanity. Since people are involved in the preparation, serving, and quality image of the establishment, it is important for the employees to feel good about themselves and good about the quality and credibility of the food service establishment.

SCENARIO—THE NASTY WAITRESS

Upon a recent visit to a seashore restaurant on a rainy day, I was saddened by the lack of concern shown our party of four by the waitress. Not only did the order take over 1 hour and 15 minutes from placement to service, but the waitress neglected her duties by ignoring our request for water or even explaining the difficulties she was experiencing in the kitchen. Her attitude lacked professionalism and, to top it off, the daily fish specials and red potatoes were served cold. Needless to say, gratuity was not considered and a return visit to a once-reputable establishment is out of the question.

The hospitality industry is a people-oriented business. Attitudes are critical in conveying a positive message. People are also a significant part of an infection-control program. Based on what we studied about how pathogenic organisms are transmitted, an infection-control program is as critical to a food and beverage operation as a positive attitude from a waitress.

SANITATION-RELATED TASKS

Before we examine some high-traffic areas, let's review certain sanitation-related tasks for service employees. Employees are required to hold cups and utensils by handles, carry multiple glasses on trays, hold glasses and dishes on the bottom, avoid stacking dishes, dispense foods like rolls and butter with tongs, and always wash their hands after potential contamination.

Let's examine some high-traffic areas:

1. The food preparation areas (main kitchen)
2. The dishwashing areas
3. Bar/lounge/food areas
4. Restaurant storage areas
5. Storage carts
6. Trays
7. Meeting rooms
8. Room service
9. The employee cafeteria

These are not all the areas that fall under food and beverage, but they are critical to guest and employee satisfaction.

The cook basically comes in contact with food and environmental surfaces necessary for the task of food preparation. But during the day he or she is also exposed to other employees and to other areas or objects that may harbor pathogenic microorganisms or potential infection. Most cooks and chefs have had sanitation training. Let's review the objectives of sanitation for cooks and chefs.

SANITATION TRAINING FOR COOKS AND CHEFS

Cooks are trained:

1. To recognize the prcblem of food-borne illness;
2. To practice good personal hygiene to avoid contaminating food;
3. To practice waste management and cleanliness to avoid pest problems;

4. To observe the time and temperature rule during all phases of food preparation; and

5. To exercise all sanitation quality control procedures.

All of these are valuable practices and objectives which are studied and learned. The difficulty lies in the implementation of these rules and procedures, because the classroom is not the same as the back of the house on a daily basis.

Kitchen evaluations have revealed, in many cases, a lack of concern for cleanliness and a chef too busy to practice good personal hygiene in between meat and fish entrees. This is all the more reason to address infection-control procedures and use high-level disinfection products in food and beverage areas.

The food service industry is experiencing a phenomenal number of food-related outbreaks of disease. It is nationally recognized that only 5 to 10 percent of food-related illnesses are reported to local environmental agencies and that the real number of illnesses is at least 25 times that reported. The FDA feels that greater efforts should be made to determine the incidences of all diarrheal and food-borne diarrheal disease.

The problem of disease transmission in food service establishments exists primarily because of a lack of barrier protection (like sneeze guards), effective personal hygiene, and proper use of sanitizing or cleaning chemicals. Certain chemicals may even be inactive against certain viruses or bacteria or may not be used according to the manufacturers' directions.

Sanitizing and *disinfecting* are two terms which are thought to mean the same thing, like so many other words in the English language. The meaning and the word's definition may not be the same; for example, the food service industry defines *sanitized* as free from disease-causing organisms, when, in fact, sterilization is the only means of removing *all* microorganisms; and sterilization is not feasible in the food service industry for surfaces and people. The next best means would be high-level disinfection chemicals which kill most organisms except spores. The microbiological definition of sanitize means only to reduce the number of microorganisms to a safe level. A safe level is vague, based on the number of organisms necessary to cause infections and the resistance of the host. Since everybody's resistance levels are different, some people are more susceptible to catching disease. Today, we are faced with many new diseases like AIDS, Hepatitis C, and Herpes II, and the same old ones, like Salmonella, Staphylococcus, and Streptococcus. Unfortunately, there are still too many unanswered questions about disease transmission. We must take steps toward reducing the risk by being prepared and using common sense.

The main concerns of food service industry have always been for time and temperature. How hot, how cold, how long, how soon, how often are all important factors which lead to many food-borne illness outbreaks. If food is prepared too soon and held at room temperature, or if stored in inadequate refrigeration, or if prepared on inadequately cleaned and sanitized surfaces or by food handlers with infected cuts, burns, or sores, and so on, problems can occur. Improper food handling, improper storage, unsanitary dishware, utensils, and equipment, and poor personal hygiene all combine to transmit food-borne illness.

The industry is constantly training employees and trying desperately to reduce the risk of disease, but unfortunately, cannot keep up with either the microbiological community or the employee turnover. Since people and food are two of the main causes that lead to disease transmission and one cannot survive without the other, it is obvious that more attention to infection-control procedures must be integrated into the ongoing employee training efforts.

Infection-control training deals with people, surfaces, and high-level disinfection product applications that can assist in greatly reducing the risk of cross-contamination and protect the employee and the guest.

TRAY CLEANING

Serving trays used by room service, for example, are exposed to many germs in hallways, freight elevators, and so on. After the dishes have been removed, are the trays thoroughly cleaned? Are they left to collect new germs? How often are trays just wiped off and stacked? More attention to little details like trays is necessary for proper disinfection and reducing cross-contamination. Trays come in contact with people as well as contaminated dishware, glassware, and utensils. The serving trays should be disinfected at least twice a day by applying a high-level disinfectant and allowing to air dry. The risk of disease transmission is greatly reduced. The application should take about 6 to 8 seconds per tray, which does not require special skills or prove to be labor intensive or costly.

BAR/LOUNGE/FOOD AREAS

Which of these sanitation procedures in cleaning lounge tables or restaurant booths would you prefer if you were the next customer?

Situation 1

The server assistant comes to the table to remove the dishes and clean the table. He or she takes a wet handiwipe carried on the soiled tray and moistens the table surface collecting some food particles, while missing others, and then proceeds to prepare the table for the next guest, handling the clean silverware after touching the cleaning cloth! *Questions:* Was the handiwipe moistened by water or had it been soaked in an effective disinfection solution? Is the food remaining in the cracks free from bacteria? Were there any nicks, cuts, or abrasions on the hands of the server assistant?

Situation 2

After your evening cocktail, the bartender takes a rag from a sink behind the counter and swishes the surface preparing for the next customer. *Questions:* Was the rag in the holding sink, wash sink, or just on a counter surface behind the bar? Was it water wet? How clean is the rag? Is there potential for infection from the moisture remaining on the counter?

These incidents do occur. The questions remain unanswered, and only if proper techniques and disinfection chemicals are utilized, are we safe from the risk of cross-contamination. The same concerns and questions apply for the employees as well as for the guests.

In all fairness to the restaurant, they are probably taking steps to ensure your safety; but this does not mean the facility is aware of infection-control procedures or is using high-level disinfectants.

Scenario

The setting is a crowded, popular Mexican eatery on a busy Saturday night.

What to Look For. If you choose to have a Margarita and munch on nachos and salsa before you are seated, keep your eyes on your cocktail glasses to be sure there is no residue from a previous customer's drink. A napkin should be placed in the basket, and tongs should be used, if available, to serve you your nacho chips. If not, a napkin should be used. Try not to reuse the same plate or container of salsa. If necessary, do not place salsa on the plate and then scrape off excess with the serving ladle. The technique of serving and removing excess from a dirty plate with a serving ladle or utensil has been observed on numerous occasions in various buffet style or self-service food bars.

When you are seated, wipe off your utensils with your napkin and be sure the table is free from food debris. The other steps and precautions must be taken by the food handlers, servers, and bartenders. The bartender has the responsibility to clean, rinse, and sanitize each glass. The food handlers and cooks have the responsibility of practicing personal hygiene and not using what appears to be contaminated food. The servers must also practice effective personal hygiene, as well as making sure the tables and utensils are properly cleaned and sanitized. The potential for cross-contamination occurs when there is either human error or misuse of sanitizing chemicals. For example, most sanitizing chemicals are chlorine deriva-tives, must be mixed with water at a specific temperature, and have a minimum required contact time to be effective. A com-mon towel used by bar staff or kitchen employees is a breeding ground for microorganisms and cross-contamination. Restau-rants have an obligation to their customers to provide not only quality service and good food, but state-of-the-art infection-control programs should be in place to greatly reduce the risk of potential disease transmission.

From July 1987 to June 1988, disease outbreaks reported to and investigated by one environmental agency, resulted in over 7,500 people being exposed to food-borne bacteria from rice, crab cakes, chicken, shredded beef, ice, cheddar melt, pizza, refried beans, vanilla milk shakes, spaghetti, turkey and stuffing, potato salad, seafood newburg, coleslaw, and water. These foods may not have been the sole source of the problem, but combined with ineffective personal hygiene and the lack of high-level disinfection, they resulted in disease transmission. Once an outbreak occurs, the damage is already done.

Food service employees are at risk from cross-infection when they receive a nick or cut in handling silverware and glassware after it has been used by a customer, transmission from uncleaned foods, and others' failure to practice good hygiene and hand washing. Table wipes that are moist are used to wipe contaminated surfaces and are then handled by a server assistant. Wouldn't you feel more comfortable knowing your cloth or handiwipe was sanitized in a high-level disinfection solution, protecting you as well as the guest?

CIRCULATION AND DISINFECTION OF UTENSILS AND GLASSWARE

Situation

All items are contaminated with a combination of food and saliva.

Solution

When silverware and glasses are removed from the table, they should be placed into a holding solution (a hospital-grade disinfectant) as quickly as possible. This will accomplish two vital functions:

1. It will keep proteinaceous material soft and easy to remove in subsequent cleaning steps.
2. The holding solution begins the disinfection process; then washing with an appropriate dishwashing solution will drastically reduce the chances of cross-infection.

Again, let's mention, that due to media attention, public awareness of infectious disease has been heightened. More and more consumers are looking more closely at their environment. The pressure on business and industry is to act, not react. Until Legionnaires' disease took its toll in Philadelphia, everyone ignored evaporative air conditioning systems. Fear of illness is on the increase and affects everyone.

THE THREE-SINK THEORY

The Wash Tank, Rinse Tank, and Sanitize Tank

Usually on a busy evening, the glassware is rapidly turned over and the need for minimum time and temperature requirements to avoid cross-contamination is often overlooked. The 2 to 3 seconds in the wash tank, the 1½ to 2 seconds dip in the rinse tank, and a 2 second dip in the sanitize tank does not come close to meeting minimum health code requirements. The liability lies with the property. If an outbreak occurs due to a lack of judgment, the problem cannot be placed on the chemical supplier. A very popular last rinse sanitizer, Beer Clean, like most, is a chlorine derivative. The manufacturer's specific directions for use said,

Note: It is a violation of federal law to use this product in a manner inconsistent with its labeling.

1. Prewash glassware.
2. Rinse with clean, cool water.
3. In the sanitizing tank, mix the contents of this package in 3 gallons of water (use test strip to assure required chlorine levels). *Immerse* glassware for at least 2 minutes or contact time specified by governing sanitary code.
4. Place glassware on rack or drainboard to air dry.

The author has observed many bartenders using the three-tank wash/rinse technique, and never has he seen one following the manufacturer's directions. The property is liable, if linked to an outbreak. Only the business suffers the consequences.

> Thousands of Americans die each year from food-borne illness and over 80 million people become ill—no one is immune [20].

Infection-control procedures are recommended in hospitals, dental offices, and dental laboratories, but implementation is still far from complete. In spite of hospital guidelines and the routine use of hospital-grade sterilization and disinfectant products, up to 40 percent of the patients admitted for some hospital service leave with a new exogenous infection (infection originating from an external source), according to the *New England Journal of Medicine*. Food and beverage services can be found in many places: health care nutrition services, employee cafeteria services, school cafeteria services, government institutions, or commercial restaurants; everyone has to eat! Food and beverage managers, chefs, or any food service worker cannot continue to assume that nothing can happen. Obviously with the continued outbreaks of Salmonella poisoning, Hepatitis A, and other related food-borne illnesses, more attention must be paid to improving the quality of cleaning and personal hygiene, than the quantity of food served.

INFECTION CONTROL FOR FOOD SERVICE OPERATIONS

The area of sanitation in dealing with food preparation and a healthy working environment is thoroughly covered in an excellent textbook by the Educational Foundation of the National Restaurant Association, *Applied Foodservice Sanitation* [21]. In considering infection-control guidelines or disinfection procedures, it must be understood that all sanitation guidelines are important when dealing with food-borne illness.

Food service sanitation is critical in preventing liabilities and must not be taken lightly. Unfortunately, since human nature is not controllable, proper procedures and guidelines become a necessity. A food- or beverage-related illness can happen anywhere. Thus sanitation may not be enough.

Example 1

Good sanitation procedures recommend handling glassware from the sides or the bottom, and not from the top or with fingers inserted inside the glassware. On a recent visit to a family breakfast establishment, not one, but three servers were carrying glassware in a contraindicated manner.

Example 2

In a popular gathering place where beverages are served, two separate cases of trench mouth and numerous throat infections were transmitted. This occurred because of the lack of proper washing and rinsing of glassware, not to mention that glasses were allowed to sit bottoms up on a moist cloth and rubber surface.

In an improperly maintained environment like this, the growth of gram-negative microorganisms spirochetes from the family *Treponemataceae* from the *T. buccale* (*Borrelia buccalis*) and *T. vincentii* groups caused the infections. Glassware, silverware, and other food service-related items have the potential for causing illnesses or infections. Because microorganisms hitchhike and grow under the right conditions, food service guidelines must address not only sanitation, but disinfection:

SANITATION + DISINFECTION = INFECTION CONTROL

The need for quality assurance must go along with the need for proper nutrition. Because different types of facilities have either central production areas or satellite feeding areas, food has to be transported, while proper temperatures are maintained. This is another reason the need for infection-control programs are important not only for the employee, but for the guests receiving the food.

Food-borne illness can spring up anywhere. A recent example is that of a major investment firm that serves employee meals in cafeterias and executive dining rooms. A Salmonella outbreak infected over 70 employees. It may have been due to contaminated food, an improperly treated food preparation surface, or an employee carrier. Improper sanitation without infection-control procedures opens the door to liabilities.

Disinfection, when applicable, is the destruction of most microorganisms when sterilization is impossible. In food service operations, sterilization is impossible. Infection control is the use of procedures that, when implemented, greatly reduce the risk of cross-contamination. Foods are impossible to disinfect, so proper sanitation guidelines for purchasing, receiving, storing, preparing, and serving foods are necessary and must be utilized. Whether it is a major outbreak of Hepatitis A or Salmonella or a minor infection or common cold, once the transmission is linked to a food service establishment the credibility suffers.

In one case, when a food handler had hepatitis and was not following a specific infection-control protocol at the time, a once profitable restaurant went from a $40,000 weekly income to less than $3,000 per week and is still suffering. Improper food service operations can be very costly to the reputation of a property. Once the damage is done, all the creative marketing in the world will not rebuild a quality reputation.

Several problems exist in the food service areas. The food itself can cause many illnesses if not properly maintained. The people working in the "back of the house," or kitchen areas, can be responsible for the transmission of diseases. The type of facility and the environmental surfaces may lead to the transmission of infections.

Risk of Disease Transmission to Food Service Employees

A. Sharp utensils cause nicks, cuts, and so on
B. Handling silverware, glasses, and so on, after use by a customer
C. Burns

(continued)

D. Bar soap

E. Common towels

F. Risk of cross-contamination of an open lesion, wound, or abrasion from environmental surfaces

G. Slippery surfaces

H. Transmission through uncleaned foods (lettuce).

Diseases Potentially Transmitted in a Food Service Environment to the Customer

Salmonella

Hepatitis A

Staphylococcus

Streptococcus

Herpes

Trench Mouth

Intestinal Flu

Risk to Guests

A. Contaminated silverware due to inadequate cleaning or sanitizing

B. Contaminated glassware or dinnerware due to exposure from organisms from the hands of employees

C. Exposure to air-borne organisms on tables, counters, and so on, promoted by air conditioning systems

D. Hepatitis risk from infected food handlers

E. Food contamination from exposure to contaminated environmental surfaces

F. Poor or nonexistent hand washing and failure to use antimicrobial soaps

G. Failure to use barrier protection by employees

People and surfaces may be addressed by implementing an effective infection-control program. The food falls under proper sanitation guidelines as addressed in sanitation textbooks. The most effective EPA registered environmental surface disinfectants usually do not address food preparation surfaces because the FDA is the government agency that monitors anything consumed or dealing with the body. However, depending upon the type of operation, certain disinfection applications are appropriate.

In daily food and beverage operations, coffee is constantly brewing and being served. In the coffee shop of one large New York City Hotel, the server's assistant, who maintained the coffee service, was observed carrying a cleaning cloth, wiping off the tables in between customers, and placing this same cloth over a pot of coffee to keep in the heat. This is certainly not a recommended technique. It could have generated the transmission of many organisms that could have led to serious liabilities, not to mention illnesses and infections.

In a recent microbiological culture study done in conjunction with a major hotel corporation, some very interesting results reinforced the need for infection-control programs. The following culture samples were taken using a Rodac plate to capture the microorganisms before and after the application of a chemical disinfection product. While the samples were taken at random in various areas of the hotel kitchen, lobby, and a guest room, our concerns here center on food service areas, and only those areas are listed.

MICROBIOLOGICAL CULTURE STUDY

Place of Sampling	Count	Organisms (Before Control Plates)
Executive Steward's office phone	TNTC*	Gram-positive, Staphylococcus

(continued)

Place of Sampling	Count	Organisms (Before Control Plates)
Executive Steward's desktop	92	Gram-positive, Diplococci
Kitchen sink handle	TNTC	Gram-positive rods, gram-negative rods
Stainless steel kitchen surface	TNTC	Gram-positive rods, gram-negative Streptococcus
Main kitchen stainless steel table top	28	Gram-positive rods
Clean knife on lobby dining area	TNTC	Gram-positive rods
Salt shaker	50	Sarcina
Dining table surface	TNTC	Gram-negative rods; gram-positive Diplococci
Dining chair	TNTC	Gram-negative rods, gram-positive rods

*TNTC denotes "too numerous to count."

The "before" plates revealed a variety of microorganisms and spore-forming rods. Staphylococcus, Streptococcus, and Diplococci can all potentially lead to some type of illness or infection under the right circumstances. Sarcina is a genus of anaerobic gram-positive cocci from the Peptococcaceae family. Whether or not it is a disease-causing bacteria is unknown.

After one application of a disinfectant product allowing for the manufacturer's suggested contact time, the test plates showed a drastic reduction of organism count.

MICROBIOLOGICAL COUNT AFTER DISINFECTION

Place of Sampling	Count	Organisms
Executive Steward's office phone	16	Gram-positive rods
Executive Steward's desktop	3	Gram-positive rods
Kitchen sink handle	23	Gram-positive rods, gram-positive cocci
Stainless steel kitchen surface	0	
Main kitchen stainless steel table top	0	
Clean knife on lobby dining area	0	
Salt shaker	0	
Dining table surface	1	Gram-positive rods
Dining chair	5	Gram-positive rods

This culture sampling revealed that even clean silverware and a freshly prepared table may harbor infection-generating organisms. This is why attention must be paid to infection control. Staphylococcus problems can arise on a daily basis if food handlers or support personnel have skin infections or open cuts, nicks, or lesions. Salmonella infections, trench mouth, mononucleosis, the common cold, and even viral diseases can be transmitted if proper sanitation and disinfection procedures are not followed.

Food Service Disinfection Procedures

Disinfection Procedures Applicable in a Food Service Operation

1. Daily, or at least routine, application of a disinfectant on food preparation surfaces, based on guidelines set by the manufacturer or the property's own infection-control program.
2. The use of a disinfectant on table surfaces in serving areas.
3. Presoaking of dishware, glassware, and silverware in an immersion-type disinfection solution prior to dish-washing.
4. The use of barrier protection:
    a. Latex gloves, when open wounds or infection exist
    b. Disposable placemats and napkins
    c. Table cloths and overlay cloths
    d. Disposable aprons worn over uniforms by all kitchen employees
    e. Hair covering
    f. Face mask when applicable for kitchen personnel
5. Periodic culture sample tests to ensure that the infection control program is working properly. These tests should be performed by an independent microbiology laboratory or by the property's infection-control consultant.

In chain food service operations, the risks of infection are intensified. Many operate 24 hours a day and are constantly seating customers, so that it is difficult to clean and reset tables or booths between parties. These types of operations need a disinfection product that can be applied with a cloth and that needs little contact time to be effective against microorganisms. Protective barriers like disposable placemats are already used in most cases. Certain kinds of restaurant tables with designs in the tops or rough surfaces also pose special problems for effective disinfection. With a rough surface or tile top, the likelihood exists that food particles and microorganisms will not be totally removed by just wiping off the table. Crusted or sticky food substances lodge in cracks and breed new microbial growth. The need for an effective table wipe or a longer contact time by the disinfectant must be observed. A popular restaurant with rough table surfaces can only damage its reputation if crusted or sticky food substances are not removed. This creates unnecessary customer aggravation, especially if an arm or elbow meets with food remnants. Wiping with plain water, without rubbing, will not remove food substances or all microorganisms that can spread infections.

Ideally, a chain operation should adopt a uniform infection-control protocol, and post the procedures at every location. Without guidelines or industry standards, liabilities may exist. If *negligence* is proven in any legal action, the property will not stand a chance of defending itself against claims of disease transmitted by food or food handlers. If an infection-control program does exist and effective disinfectant products are being used and monitored, liabilities should, in most cases, be reduced.

Many food service operations at one time or another have known about illnesses caused by tainted food or improper preparation, but have been fortunate enough not to be legally challenged. This luck does not eliminate the need for effective steps to prevent or reduce the risk of recurrence. The need exists now, more than ever before, to properly address infection control. The 1980s will be known as the "decade of new diseases" if we continue to tolerate improper food service techniques. You do not want your facility to be known as the first restaurant to transmit the AIDS virus to a customer. A regular regimen of precautions is the best defense. Diseases which did not exist 15 years ago are now making the need for infection-control awareness and disinfection procedures a necessary part of any food service operation.

Product Application: Food Service Areas

1. Types of disinfectants
   a. Spray-aerosol/nonaerosol pump
   b. Multipurpose bulk liquid
   c. Disposable wipes
   d. Antimicrobial cleaning lotion
   e. Drain cleaner/sanitizer concentrate
2. Applications
   a. All kitchen work surfaces—sinks, table tops, and so on. Daily or routinely, depending upon infection control protocol
   b. Holding tanks (kitchens, lounges, counters)
   c. Additive for mopping floors
   d. Employee hand-washing protection
   e. Presoak prior to warewashing

Product Directions: Food Service Areas

Remember, disinfection is different from sanitizing. Disinfectants are formulated to totally eliminate viral and bacteriological organisms, except spores. Sanitizers are only meant to reduce the count of microorganisms to what is considered a "safe" level. Follow these instructions:

(continued)

1. All food products must be removed or carefully covered and protected.

2. To preclean surface, spray until wet, then dry with tissue, paper towel, or cloth.

3. To disinfect, hold the spray nozzle 6 to 8 inches from the precleaned surface. Spray 2 to 4 seconds, or until the surface is covered with mist. Allow 10 minutes contact time.

4. Rinse all food contact surfaces with potable water before reuse.

Infection-Control Protocol General Recommendations

Food Service Establishments

Barrier protection for food handlers

Antimicrobial soaps

High-level disinfection product applications —routinely

OSHA compliance programs for employees

On-site culture samples

Proper hand washing techniques

Food certification test for all managers and food handlers

Ongoing educational and training programs on infection control

SUMMARY

1. In a hotel, proper food service sanitation and disinfection can help create a high quality image and attract and keep business.

2. Food service sanitation procedures and chemicals are doing an adequate job, but may not be effective enough to completely eliminate the risk of cross-infection.

3. All food service workers should use antimicrobial soap, hand protection, and other protective barriers if they have a cold or any other infection.

4. Food service areas can either be disinfected daily or routinely during the week depending upon the type of operation and the efficacy of the product used for disinfection.

5. Food and beverage directors and all personnel should be motivated to act toward establishing quality standards of infection-control procedures and using state-of-the-art high-level disinfection products wherever applicable in specific food service operations.

REVIEW EXERCISES

1. Keeping customer loyalty is most often the responsibility of:
   a. housekeeping
   b. corporate
   c. food and beverage

2. The lodging and hospitality industry began to show concern after the outbreak of:
   a. hepatitis
   b. AIDS
   c. Legionnaires

3. Food and beverage activities parallel those of:
   a. hospitals
   b. Wendy's
   c. dental labs

4. Hepatitis A can be transmitted by:
   a. food handlers
   b. paper cut
   c. blood

5. The serving trays used by room service are usually:
   a. stacked
   b. disinfected
   c. disposable

6. Food and beverage directors and personnel should be motivated to:
   a. act "versus" react
   b. avoid work
   c. hire only college graduates

7. A properly implemented infection-control program would greatly reduce the risk of cross-contamination.

   True or False?

8. In food service areas if a disinfectant is used in between food preparation, what is the most important step in the instruction?

8

Marketing Infection Control

KEY CONCEPTS

Perception Is Reality	**Reach the Customer**
Public Awareness	**Enhance your Image**
Positive Marketing Steps	

While outbreaks of disease are not occurring every day in the hospitality industry, it is nevertheless the perception of the traveling public that disease can be acquired in hotels, motels, and restaurants. Currently, the public's fears are considerably greater than the actual risks. From a marketing standpoint, facilities offering infection-control programs will gain a significant competitive advantage. The marketing value of such a program, however, depends upon public awareness. Favorable public response has resulted in other business situations where infection-control programs have been instituted and publicized.

One way of letting guests know about your program is the infection-control checklist. A copy of a checklist enumerating all the steps taken to prepare for a new guest's arrival should be left in the guest room. In this way, the arriving guest is assured that his or her room has been prepared in accordance with the highest standards available.

Another innovative marketing tool would be a direct mail campaign to a select group of recent guests, offering a discount on the next visit and explaining the new infection-control program. This would bring more guests back for a return visit to the same location, or other locations in a large chain, while at the same time attracting new guests through word-of-mouth advertising.

As a service industry, we must treat perception as reality, act to create a standard of excellence in infection control, and market our new infection-control procedures. The public will respond favorably to a policy that speaks to this concern and allays their fears.

The public responds favorably to new gimmicks, like fast food meal promotions, specialty items for dessert, or do-it-yourself Cajun cooking, for example. In hotels, guests appreciate amenities like free coffee and a paper, a courteous staff, and a pleasant environment convenient for business; hotels and restaurants compete for market share like any other businesses. Sales are generated by offering a new innovative product or service or stealing sales from the competition. The most positive marketing step to generate new business is to be first; leaders always benefit in creating new business.

Instituting a program of high-level disinfection procedures, without making the customer aware of them, is not sufficient. Therefore, it is mandatory that a parallel marketing program accompany the infection-control or disinfection policy established by the property.

REACHING THE CUSTOMER

There are three basic customer groups with which a property needs to communicate in order to achieve the dual objective of acquiring new patrons and gaining repeat business. The first group is made up of former patrons who have been customers within the last six months. The second group is current patrons—registered guests or frequent diners. The third group, the future visitors to the area, who have never been to the property before now.

MARKETING IDEAS: LODGING ESTABLISHMENTS

Group 1

Names and addresses of recent guests are on record so that former patrons can be selected at random and sent a brochure explaining the new high-level disinfection procedures. The brochure can be accompanied by a coupon offering a reduced room rate or other discounts on a return visit.

Group 2

Present guests may be presented a brochure at check-in or a checklist may be placed in the room designed to alert the guest about your program. Special amenities may be provided containing small containers of surface disinfectant, antimicrobial soap, and disposable towelettes.

Group 3

New patrons will be the most difficult to reach, because they are unknown. However, if your property advertises in local magazines or road club publications, it will not be difficult to publicize your infection-control program, designed to create a healthier environment for the guest. Word-of-mouth advertising will undoubtedly occur once your patrons know about the steps you have taken to ensure their comfort and health during business or vacation travel.

Guest Room Checklist

( ) Sleeping area vacuumed

( ) Carpets disinfected routinely

( ) Floors, walls, and baseboards dust-free

( ) Wastebaskets emptied, wiped clean, and disinfected

( ) Drapes in place, work properly, and disinfected routinely

( ) Light fixtures cleaned and in working order

( ) Bed freshly made and smooth (blankets, pillows, and bedspreads disinfected routinely)

( ) T.V. in good working order

( ) Room amenities stocked to standards

( ) Mirror and windows cleaned

( ) Sink and related bathroom surfaces cleaned and then disinfected for your use

( ) Your room has been properly disinfected and prepared to make your visit healthier and more enjoyable.

MARKETING IDEAS: RESTAURANTS

All three customer groups are combined when dealing with food service facilities. Your old and current customers come back because the atmosphere, service, and quality of food justifies a return visit. New customers will either hear of your property from others or see advertising that may be done locally.

It is more difficult for a restaurant to market its infection-control program without creating additional liability problems. Food-related infections cannot be totally eliminated, since we cannot adequately disinfect meats, fish, poultry, and vegetables. Certain advantages exist, for the employees, in using antimicrobial soap and proper barrier protection. The surfaces you disinfect greatly reduce the risk of cross-infection, but cannot totally eliminate all the microorganisms present in the food itself. Your marketing effort, therefore, is limited to the restroom facilities, where a nicely mounted plaque or framed certificate will describe your disinfection procedures. A certificate of attendance at an infection-control seminar or continuing education course should be obtained and placed near your operating license. Recently, it was suggested that high-level disinfectants or specialty items pertaining to infection control could be placed in a vending machine and positioned in restrooms or other traffic areas. This could generate additional revenues for the establishments already using these items to protect their staff and guests.

The marketing of infection control is entirely up to the specific lodging and food service facility. The main objective is to do something to protect customers and enhance your service. Our environment and atmosphere are only as safe and as healthy as we attempt to make them. By learning about disinfection and how to deal with high-risk employees, you are actively participating in your own welfare. You are helping to create a standard that no longer ignores the possibility of cross-infection. You are helping to allay the fears of a public already concerned and aware of infectious disease.

Infection control is highly exploitable from the standpoint of marketing and public relations. Keep in mind the story of the two hikers who encountered a large grizzly bear on a trail. One hiker immediately began changing from his heavy hiking boots into a pair of running shoes he was carrying. The other hiker looked in amazement and exclaimed, "Hey, you can't outrun that bear." The first hiker quickly completed the shoe change and responded, "I don't have to outrun the bear; I just have to outrun you!"

In many ways this parallels the capability of members of the lodging and hospitality industries to attain a slight but significant competitive advantage. If you are prepared for the unexpected, in most cases you will have an edge on your competitors. By implementing infection-control programs and using state-of-the-art disinfection chemicals, you will be prepared and will create a new industry standard of excellence.

A service industry cannot afford to be reactive about a problem once the consumer perceives that it exists. The future belongs to those who care enough to show concern and not wait for a policy or a written directive.

Recently, a major hotel corporation chain started a campaign called **DIRFT**, which stands for **DO IT RIGHT THE FIRST TIME**. This public-relations program has meaning for the employees and customers, but more importantly should reflect a new attitude for the 1990s. **DO IT RIGHT THE FIRST TIME** by having an infection-control training policy to reduce the property's liabilities and greatly reduce the risk of disease transmission.

SUMMARY

1. The public perceives risks from contagious diseases because the media constantly addresses AIDS, hepatitis, Legionnaires, and other infectious outbreaks.

2. The industry can no longer avoid dealing with the topic of infection control.

3. If addressed properly, infection control can be positively marketed to your customers. The safety and health of everyone should be of concern to any employer.

4. A disinfection program and public awareness of it can create a competitive advantage for a property that acts rather than reacting.

REVIEW EXERCISES

1. An infection-control program is only valuable if it is kept a secret.

   True or False

2. The public will respond favorably if policies exist for their benefit.

   True or False

3. What are the three basic customer groups to address in order to gain repeat or new business?

4. If a guest room checklist is utilized by a lodging establishment, is it good marketing to inform the guest about disinfection procedures?

   Yes or No

5. Food handler certification and continuing education about infection control will generate credibility.

   True or False

OSHA Employee Compliance Training

KEY CONCEPTS

Employee Protection
The Right to Know Law
Hazard Communication
   Standard

Employee Training
Material Safety Data
   Sheets (MSDS)

In May 1989, an OSHA inspector visited a hotel property in Long Island, New York, to determine whether OSHA standards were being followed. When an inspector enters a property, an opening conference is arranged between a representative from management and the employees' union (if a union is present) or a representative selected to participate by the employees. In the opening conference, the OSHA inspector asks a few basic questions.

1. Do you have OSHA poster 2203 posted on the employee bulletin board?
2. Are you keeping records of work-related injuries and illnesses on OSHA Form 200?
3. When do you normally post Form 200?

4. Have your employees been informed and trained in accordance with the Hazard Communication Standard?

5. May I see your written training programs?

6. Do you have a fire protection and prevention plan available?

These opening questions are basically standard. Others may also be included. Depending upon the answers, the property may be subject to a *wall-to-wall* OSHA inspection.

OSHA INSPECTIONS

The unsuspecting property on Long Island, as described on pages 137 and 138, either did not correctly respond to the initial questions or did not have the requested information and was subsequently subjected to a six-day inspection, during which the property was cited for numerous violations with fines totaling approximately $14,000.00. The fines were reduced for the capability to immediately abate certain violations, but the property still faced $6,000.00 in fines. OSHA fines are not considered a deductible business expense.

OSHA has targeted the hotel, motel, and restaurant industry for inspections because of repeated incidences which have been dangerous and life-threatening to employees. Based on Public Law 91-596, OSHA was established in 1970 for the protection of employees. Numerous standards and regulations have been proposed for employee safety in both manufacturing and nonmanufacturing settings since OSHA was formed. Employees under the Right to Know Act are required to be informed and trained on specific OSHA standards.

Hotels, motels, and restaurants must be aware of the areas OSHA targets in the event of an inspection visit. Remember, OSHA's only concern is for employees' safety and awareness of how to avoid hazards in the workplace. The hazard communication standard, which requires all employers to train employees on chemicals in the workplace, is the primary concern for hotels, motels, and restaurants. Why? Because most sanitation, disinfection, and cleaning products are registered with the Environmental Protection Agency and considered hazardous by OSHA. Over 2,000 chemicals are on the OSHA list—insecticides, bleach, ammonia, quaternary ammonium compounds, alcohol, phenols, formaldehyde, glutaraldehydes, and the list continues. All of these chemicals are found in formulas which hotels, motels, and restaurants use every day for cleaning, sanitizing, and disinfecting surfaces. A question to ask would be: Are your employees aware of the use, handling, and hazards associated with these products? That's what OSHA is going to find out when conducting an inspection.

There are some basic areas of the hazard communication standard which must be addressed. First, do you (the property) have a written Hazard Communication Program? Second, do

HAZARD COMMUNICATION PROGRAM

Employee Handout

The Employee Right-to-Know

OSHA Hazard Communication Standard (29 CRF 1910.1200)

The law requires that chemical manufacturers and importers...

- evaluate products and determine whether there are any physical or health hazards associated with using them.
- communicate their findings via labels and Material Safety Data Sheets for each product they manufacture.

The law requires that your employer...

- establish a written Hazard Communication Program that explains exactly how he is going to inform you and your fellow workers about hazards and how to handle them. You should be able to see this program at any time.
- label products appropriately.
- obtain Material Safe Data Sheets (MSDS's) for all products with physical or health hazards. These documents should be kept in a place where you can easily refer to them.
- train you to identify and deal with hazardous materials and make you aware of any new hazards introduced into your work area.

Before you start any job, YOU should...

- read labels and MSDS documents.
- identify any hazardous materials and get the proper equipment to work with them safely. Never mix chemicals together unless specifically instructed to do so.
- always use proper techniques to perform your tasks - and be familiar with emergency procedures.
- ask your supervisor when you have any questions.

Everyone - government, manufacturers, your employer - everyone wants you to be safe. That's why these laws were developed. But your safety is up to YOU. So take advantage of the law. Inform yourself, learn how to use chemical products safely, and be sure to exercise the little extra care that's called for.

This is to certify that the provisions of the federal Hazard Communications Standard have been explained to me, and that I have been told where to obtain copies of MSDS sheets.

_____ _____ _____
Employee signature   Location   Date

Figure 9.1 Sample Hazard Communication Program form.

you receive and properly make available Material Safety Data Sheets? Third, have your employees been trained? Fourth, do your employees have access to your Hazard Communication Program?

The hazard communication written program must include the specific methods that are used to achieve compliance with the requirements of the Hazard Communication Standard (29CFR 1910 1200) (see the following sample program).

Note: Laboratories and agricultural employers do not have to prepare written programs. However, the department recommends that these employers prepare a written program to provide a basis for follow-up, evaluation, and improvement of their hazard communication program.

Sample Written Hazard Communication Program

1. Company Policy

   To ensure that information about the dangers of all hazardous chemicals used by (name of company) are known by all affected employees, the following hazardous information program has been established:

   All work units of the company will participate in the hazard communication program. This written program will be available in the (location) for review by any interested employee.

2. Container Labeling

   The (person/position) will verify that all containers received for use will be clearly labeled as to the contents, note the appropriate hazard warning, and list the name and address of the manufacturer.

   The (person/position) in each section will ensure that all secondary containers are labeled with either

   (continued)

an extra copy of the original manufacturer's label or with labels that have the identity and the appropriate hazard warning. For help with labeling, see (per-son/position).

Note: If written alternatives to in-plant container are used, add a description of the system used.

The (person/position) will review the company labeling procedures every (time period) and update as required.

3. Material Safety Data Sheets (MSDS)

The (person/position) is responsible for establishing and monitoring the company MSDS program. He/she will make sure procedures are developed to obtain the necessary MSDSs and will review incoming MSDSs for new or significant health and safety information. He/she will see that any new information is passed on to affected employees.

Copies of MSDSs for all hazardous chemicals in use will be kept in (location).

MSDSs will be available to all employees during each work shift. If a MSDS is not available, immediately contact (person/position).

Note: If an alternative to material safety data sheets is used, provide a description of the format.

4. Employee Training and Information

The (person/position) is responsible for the company employee training program. He/she will ensure that all program elements specified below are carried out.

Prior to starting work, each new employee of (name of company) will attend a health and safety orientation that includes the following information and training:

(continued)

- An overview of the requirements contained in the Hazard Communication Standard
- Hazardous chemicals present at his/her workplace
- Physical and health risks of the hazardous chemicals
- The symptoms of overexposure
- How to determine the presence or release of hazardous chemicals in his/her work area
- How to reduce or prevent exposure to hazardous chemicals through use of control procedures, work practices, and personal protective equipment
- Steps the company has taken to reduce or prevent exposure to hazardous chemicals
- Procedures to follow if employees are overexposed to hazardous chemicals
- How to read labels and review MSDSs to obtain hazard information
- Location of the MSDS file and written hazard communication program

Prior to introducing a new chemical hazard into any section of this company, each employee in that section will be given information and training as outlined above for the new chemical hazard.

5. Hazardous Nonroutine Tasks

Periodically, employees are required to perform hazardous nonroutine tasks. Some examples of nonroutine tasks are: confined space entry, tank cleaning, and painting reactor vessels. Prior to starting work on such projects, each affected employee will be given information by the (person/position) about the hazardous chemicals he or she may encounter during such an activity. This information will include specific chemical hazards, protective and safety measures the employee can use, and steps the company is using to

(continued)

reduce the hazards, including ventilation, respirators, presence of another employee, and emergency procedures.

6. Informing Contractors

It is the responsibility of (person/position/department/etc.) to provide contractors with information about hazardous chemicals their employees may be exposed to on a jobsite and suggested precautions for the contractor's employees.

The following option is recommended for your program: contractors will be contacted before work is started to gather and distribute information concerning any chemical hazard that they may bring to our workplace.

7. List of Hazardous Chemicals

The following is a list of all known hazardous chemicals used by our employees. Further information on each chemical may be obtained by reviewing MSDSs located at (location).

MSDS Identity

(Here's where you put the chemical list developed during the inventory. Arrange this list so that you are able to cross-reference it with your MSDS file and the labels on your containers.)

The next major issue deals with the Material Safety Data Sheet (MSDS) (Figures 9.2 and 9.3). The MSDS is designed to inform employees about any hazards found in a chemical product used in the workplace. The MSDS must be readily accessible to all employees. If the MSDS log is kept locked in the fire safety director's office, it is not considered to be accessible. The best place for 24-hour accessibility by employees must be determined by each property. It is recommended that additional MSDS copies be kept where all chemicals are stored or used as well as in the main log.

MATERIAL SAFETY DATA SHEET

This form may be used to comply with OSHA's Hazard Communication Standard, 29 CFR 1920.1200. To be valid, all information required by § 1910.1200(g) of the Standard must appear on this form. Consult the Standard for specific requirements. Note: Blank spaces are not permitted. If any item is not applicable, or no information is available, the space must be marked to indicate that.

IDENTITY (As used on Label and List)

Section I

Manufacturer's name	Emergency Telephone Number
Address (number, street, city, state and ZIP code)	Telephone Number for Information
	Date Prepared
	Signature of Preparer (optional)

Section II - Hazardous Ingredients/Identity Information

Hazardous Components (Specific Chemical Identity/Common Name(s)	OSHA PEL	ACGIH TLV	Other limits Recommended	%

Section III - Physical/Chemical Characteristics

Boiling Point	Specific Gravity ($H_2O = 1$)
Vapor Pressure (mm Hg.)	Melting Point
Vapor Density (AIR = 1)	Evaporation Rate (Butyl Acetate = 1)
Solubility in Water	
Appearance and Odor	

Section IV - Fire and Explosion Hazard Data

Flash Point (Method Used)	Flammable Limits	LEL	UEL
Extinguishing Media			

Special Fire Fighting Procedures

Unusual Fire and Explosion Hazards

Based on Draft of OSHA 174, September 1985.
Replaces obsolete OSHA form 20 MSDS

Figure 9.2. First page of sample Material Safety Data Sheet.

Section V - Reactivity Data

Stability	Unstable		Conditions to Avoid
	Stable		

Incompatibility (Materials to Avoid)

Hazardous Decomposition or Byproducts

Hazardous Polymerization	May Occur		Conditions to Avoid
	Will Not Occur		

Section VI - Health Hazard Data

Routes of Entry:	Inhalation?	Skin?	Ingestion?

Target Organs:
Health Hazards (Acute and Chronic)

Carcinogenicity:	NTP?	IARC Monographs?	OSHA Regulated?

Signs and Symptoms of Exposure

Medical Conditions Generally Aggravated by Exposure

Emergency and First Aid Procedures

Section VII - Precautions for Safe Handling and Use

Steps to Be Taken in Case Material is Released or Spilled

Waste Disposal Method

Precautions to Be Taken in Handling and Storing

Other Precautions

Section VIII - Control Measures

Respiratory Protection (Specify Types)

Ventilation	Local Exhaust	Special
	Mechanical (General)	Other
Protective Gloves		Eye Protection

Other Protective Clothing or Equipment

Work/Hygiene/Maintenance Practices

Figure 9.3. Second page of sample Material Safety Data Sheet.

Material Safety Data Sheets

Understanding the MSDS Form

The MSDS contains information about the hazardous chemical(s) found in a product or material being used in the workplace. The form used for an MSDS is in compliance with OSHA's Hazard Communication Standard, 29 CFR 1910.1200. In order to be valid, every hazardous chemical an employer uses must be made available on an MSDS.

An MSDS must be readily accessible to employees in the workplace. No blank spaces are permitted on an MSDS. If you do not know if information is available (cannot find it through a variety of sources), use UNK (unknown) in the space. If information is not applicable to the material, write N.A. in the space.

The MSDS forms do not represent all of the chemicals found for every material. Employers are required to update this section with MSDSs from the manufacturer for each new hazardous chemical that enters the workplace.

Below is an explanation of what information needs to be completed in each section of the preceding MSDS.

Identity

This section identifies the most common materials used in the workplace. The information recorded here would be used on the corresponding label for the individual product. If the employer feels the information found on the MSDS form corresponds with the material(s) the workplace is using, the brandname of the product can be entered here.

Section I

Name, address, and phone number of the MSDS preparer, distributor, or manufacturer of your brand name

(continued)

product is indicated here. The date the MSDS was prepared is also indicated in this section.

Section II   Hazardous Ingredients/Identity Information

This section asks for the hazardous components of the material identified in the **IDENTITY** section. A brief description to identify the material is listed also.

- **OSHA PEL:** Defines the permissible exposure level of the chemical.

- **ACGIH TLV:** Defines the American Conference of Governmental Industrial Hygienists Threshold Limit Value. TLV means the air-borne concentration of the substance which represents conditions under which it is believed nearly all workers may be repeatedly exposed day after day without adverse effects.

SECTION III   Physical/Chemical Characteristics

From the hazardous components identified in **SECTION II,** information can be obtained on the boiling point of the chemicals, appearance, melting point, solubility in water, vapor pressure, and density (see Glossary of Terms for the definitions of these characteristics).

SECTION IV   Fire and Explosion Hazard Data

This section contains information on the flash point of the chemical, how to extinguish a fire involving the chemical, and unusual hazards associated with this chemical.

SECTION V   Reactivity Data

This will give the worker information that can aid in the storage and handling of the chemical.

- **STABILITY:** This is how a chemical will react in its pure state when it self-reacts under conditions of shock, pressure, or temperature.

- **INCOMPATIBILITY:** How other materials or contaminants in which the hazardous chemical may

(continued)

come in contact with will produce a reaction.

- **HAZARDOUS DECOMPOSITION PRODUCTS:** Hazardous chemicals may produce dangerous amounts by burning, heating or oxidizing.
- **HAZARDOUS POLYMERIZATION:** This takes place when a chemical cures or hardens releasing large amounts of energy. The catalyst to cause this may be from heat, temperature, sunlight, etc.

SECTION VI Health Hazard Data

Information here must note the target organs that are affected. This information is required for the labeling.

- **ROUTES OF ENTRY:** The potential routes of exposure of the chemical during normal use may be ingestion, inhalation, absorption or contact.
- **CARCINOGENICITY:** If the chemical is found in one or more of the following periodicals, place a check next to the name in which the chemical appears.
- **NTP:** National Toxicology Program report
- **IARC MONOGRAPHS:** International Agency for Research on Cancer
- **OSHA:** Does OSHA classify this chemical as a potential carcinogen?

SECTION VII Precautions for Safe Handling and Use

- **IN THE EVENT OF A SPILL:** List here what is to be done in the event of a spill or leak.
- **WASTE DISPOSAL METHOD:** How to dispose of hazardous solids and liquids. How to properly clean up after an accidental spill.
- **PRECAUTION TO BE TAKEN:** Describes storage and handling so as not to cause a hazardous reaction.

(continued)

SECTION VIII   Control Measures

- **RESPIRATORY PROTECTION:** List the type of protective equipment, type of ventilation (1) and precautions to be used when handling this material or when accidentally spilled.

- **PROTECTIVE GLOVES:** Give the type of gloves needed to handle the hazardous material or indicate if protection is needed.

- **EYE PROTECTION:** List goggles or face shield protection if needed.

- **VENTILATION:** Local exhaust is done through equipment that captures fumes at the source. Mechanical would imply all use areas.

- **WORK/HYGIENE/MAINTENANCE PRACTICES:** Notes what personal hygiene steps the employee must take when handling this material.

Material Safety Data Sheet Checklist

You must ensure that each MSDS contains the following information:

1. Product or chemical identity used on the label.   _____

2. Manufacturer's name and address.   _____

3. Chemical and common names of each hazardous ingredient.   _____

4. Name, address, and phone number for hazard and emergency information.   _____

5. Preparation or revision date.   _____

6. The hazardous chemical's physical and chemical characteristics, such as vapor pressure and flashpoint.   _____

(continued)

7. Physical hazards, including the potential for fire, explosion, and reactivity. _____

8. Known health hazards. _____

9. OSHA permissible exposure limit (PEL), ACGIH threshold limit value (TLV) or other exposure limits. _____

10. Emergency and first-aid procedures. _____

11. Whether OSHA, NTP or IARC lists the ingredient as a carcinogen. _____

12. Precautions for safe handling and use. _____

13. Control measures such as engineering controls, work practices, hygienic practices or personal protective equipment required. _____

14. Primary routes of entry. _____

15. Procedures for spills, leaks, and clean-up. _____

If your property can respond positively to the MSDS checklist, you will avoid OSHA citations.

Another area seriously looked into by OSHA inspectors is the fire safety and prevention programs for each property. If your facility has a fire brigade, make sure all employees are trained to use the equipment. Get the fire department to do the training and provide written evidence to show that your employees have completed the necessary training on handling equipment and preventing a fire from causing damage or loss of life.

The fire protection checklist following contains all the key areas covered by OSHA.

Fire Protection Checklist for Hotels/Motels

OK	Action Needed	
____	____	1. Emergency plan developed and discussed with employees?
____	____	2. Emergency drills conducted at least annually?
____	____	3. Employee emergency alarms distinctive, operating properly?
____	____	4. Smoke detectors, alarms in good working order?
____	____	5. Water sprinkler systems in good condition?
____	____	6. All exits clearly marked and unobstructed?
____	____	7. All exits and exit signs appropriately illuminated?
____	____	8. Sufficient exit capacity available for occupancy?
____	____	9. Stairways in good condition with appropriate railings?
____	____	10. Fire doors installed as required and in proper operating condition?
____	____	11. Fire walls located as required?
____	____	12. Flammable materials stored in proper containers?
____	____	13. "No Smoking" areas clearly marked?
____	____	14. Portable fire extinguishers readily accessible, inspected monthly, recharged regularly?
____	____	15. Employees taught to use extinguishers?
____	____	16. Local fire department aware of hotel facilities and fire protection systems?

Training is a key for all employees. When OSHA inspectors visit hotels, motels, restaurants, nursing homes, etc., they talk with employees and ask some basic questions: Have you been trained on the Hazard Communication Standard? If so, did you learn anything?

The training programs must have a means of being measured. More than a registration form is required, because questions will be asked. A training test for employees follows.

J. D. Group, Inc., Training Test for Employees

1. Products used must have a label explaining hazards. True or False?

2. Our written safety and hazard communication program is located _____.

3. The MSDS (Material Safety Data Sheets) explain about the chemicals we use.

   True or False?

4. I have read the *OSHA Job Safety ad Health Protection* bulletin form 2203 on the employee bulletin board. True or False?

5. We have had employee training on:
   a. Hazard Communication
   b. The Right to Know Law
   c. Fire Safety
   d. All of the above.

6. The MSDS form has eight (VIII) sections covering information on hazardous chemicals.

   True or False?

7. Our training program covered emergency and First Aid procedures.

   True or False?

(continued)

8. The "Exit" signs are clearly marked.
   True or False?
9. Emergency exits (doors) are never locked or blocked.
   True or False?
10. OSHA is only concerned about:
    a. The kitchen
    b. Danger
    c. MSDS
    d. The employee

OSHA is becoming more aggressive in targeting non-manufacturing sector businesses. Hotels, motels, and restaurants are identified as dealing in hazardous chemicals, having had problems with fires resulting in the loss of life, and in general, having shown a lack of employee training. If you want to avoid inspections, citations, and costly fines, The J.D. Group Inc., Infection Control Training Center specializes in OSHA Employee Safety/Compliance Training. The company provides in-house training sessions to cover all shifts and a complete manual for ongoing programs. The company also provides a mock walk-through inspection service to identify and correct potential violations. OSHA provides this service at no charge, but they tell you up front, if you have a walk-through done by an OSHA inspector, they will be back to be sure that everything identified has been abated. If not, you are fined. The training checklist shown is actually used by OSHA inspectors. If your property completes all the necessary training requirements listed, more than likely you will avoid fines in this area.

Training Checklist

	Complete	Incomplete
1. Established a thorough training program.	_____	_____
2. Identified employees who need training.	_____	_____
3. Training program ensures that new employees are trained before their first assignment.	_____	_____
4. Informed employees of the specific information and training requirements of the Hazard Communication Standard.	_____	_____
5. Informed employees of the standard, and their rights under the law.	_____	_____
6. Informed employees of our written program and training requirements.	_____	_____
7. Informed employees of the different types of chemicals and the hazards associated with them.	_____	_____
8. Informed employees of specific hazards of the chemicals and processes they work with and their proper use and handling.	_____	_____

(continued)

9. Informed employees of the hazards associated with performing non-routine tasks.   _____   _____

10. Employees know how to detect the presence or release of hazardous chemicals in the workplace.   _____   _____

11. Trained employees in the use of proper work practices, personal protective equipment and clothing, and other controls to reduce or eliminate their exposure to the chemicals in their work areas.   _____   _____

12. Trained employees in emergency and first-aid procedures and signs of overexposure.   _____   _____

13. Listed all the hazardous chemicals in our workplace.   _____   _____

14. Employees know when and how to update our hazardous chemical list.   _____   _____

15. Obtained or developed a material safety data sheet for each hazardous chemical in the workplace.   _____   _____

16. Explained how to use an MSDS.   _____   _____

17. Informed employees of the list of hazardous chemicals and MSDSs and where they are located.   _____   _____

18. Explained labels and their warnings to employees.   _____   _____

(continued)

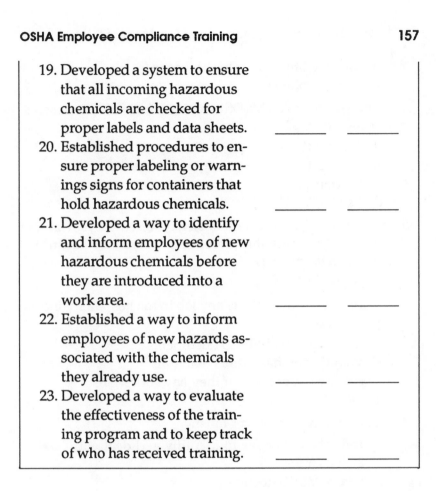

19. Developed a system to ensure that all incoming hazardous chemicals are checked for proper labels and data sheets. _____ _____

20. Established procedures to ensure proper labeling or warnings signs for containers that hold hazardous chemicals. _____ _____

21. Developed a way to identify and inform employees of new hazardous chemicals before they are introduced into a work area. _____ _____

22. Established a way to inform employees of new hazards associated with the chemicals they already use. _____ _____

23. Developed a way to evaluate the effectiveness of the training program and to keep track of who has received training. _____ _____

REVIEW QUESTIONS

1. OSHA inspections occur if an employee complains about a work related hazard.

   True or False?

2. Hotels, motels, and resturants are required by law to have a written hazard communication program.

   True or False?

3. Material Safety Data Sheets are used to:

   a. label products

    b. identify physical or health hazards

    c. train employees

4. Which section of an MSDS contains information on hazardous ingredients?

    a. Section II

    b. Section I

    c. Section VI

    d. Section V

5. A hotel, motel, or resturant must have an employee training program to detect the presence or release of hazardous chemicals in the workplace.

True or False?

6. Before an employee starts any job in the hospitality industry they should:

    a. read labels and MSDS documents

    b. identify any hazardous materials

    c. ask their supervisor if they have questions

    d. all of the above

7. The hospitality employer must:

    a. train the employee to identifiy and deal with hazardous materials

    b. secure MSDS documents

    c. post OSHA form 2203

    d. all of the above

Review Self-test

1. Which of the following statements about infection control is true?
    a. Infection-control measures must be perfect to have an effective program.
    b. Infection-control is a matter of numbers, and any step which reduces the numbers of organisms reduces the likelihood of disease transmisson.
    c. Infection-control practices currently used in restaurants always utilize the latest developments in methods and materials.
2. Hepatitus A organisms are most likely to be found in which of the following?
    a. Food contaminated by blood or other body fluids
    b. Food contaminated by sneezing or coughing
    c. Food which has been inadequately refrigerated
3. Which of the following is an example of sanitation?
    a. Application of an EPA approved disinfectant to a food preparation counter top immediately upon completion of its use
    b. Boiling silverware
    c. Cleaning a counter top after use
    d. Use of gloves by food handlers

4. Of the following methods of disinfectant product application, which is the most acceptable?

   a. Application of an EPA approved disinfectant to a soiled counter top immediately after completion of its use

   b. Thorough cleaning of a used counter top followed by application of an EPA approved disinfectant and vigorous drying of the product by wiping

   c. Thorough cleaning of a used counter top followed by application of an EPA approved disinfectant and allowing it to air dry

   d. Pouring boiling water over the counter top

5. Which of the following best describes the meaning of a high-level disinfectant?

   a. A material that kills all organisms of all types

   b. A material that kills Staphylococcus and Streptococcus

   c. A material that kills Staphylococcus, Streptococcus, and Pseudomonas

   d. A material that kills organisms which are resistant to being killed such as the mycobacterium tuberculosis but does not kill the most resistant spore-forming organisms

6. Of the following conditions found in food service establishments, the one most likely to cause disease transmission is

   a. Silverware that is inadequately cleaned allowing food to remain

   b. A food handler with athlete's foot

   c. Food contaminated by human waste

   d. A counter top inadequately disinfected

7. A food preparer cuts his or her finger during a busy time of the day. Which is the most appropriate action for this person to take?

   a. Continue working.

   b. Put on a bandage at the first opportunity and resume working.

   c. Stop immediately, put on a bandage, and resume working.

   d. Stop immediately, leave the food preparation area, and seek the necessary medical attention. Do not resume work until authorized to do so and after the necessary barriers in the form of bandages and gloves are in place. *Any* blood in the food preparation area must be *thoroughly* cleaned and a high-level EPA disinfectant used according to the manufacturers' specifications.

8. Food service employees who prepare food are required to wash their hands. Which best describes a proper handwashing technique?

   a. Surgical type scrubing using antimicrobial soap lasting 3 to 5 minutes and using a brush

   b. After removing all jewelry, scrubbing about 30 to 60 seconds total, involving three repetitions of lathering, and rinsing with an antimicrobial soap from a dispenser; drying hands on disposable paper towels

   c. Washing hands with bar soap and drying with cloth towel that is reused for economy

   d. Rinse hands and wipe on apron

9. After a kitchen is closed for the day, which best describes the application of a disinfectant?

   a. Apply disinfectant to surface and wipe dry

   b. Scrub surface with disinfectant containing a surfactant (cleaning agent) or clean thoroughly with another cleaner followed by application of the disinfectant and allow to air dry

   c. Apply disinfectant to the food preparation areas only and wipe dry

10. What best describes the objective of an infection-control protocol?

   a. To sanitize surfaces

   b. To immunize food handlers

    c. To use barriers such as gloves

    d. To reduce microorganisms to the lowest possible number, prevent cross-contamination, and break the circle of infection

11. What best describes the actions that should be taken if a food handler is thought to have a contagious disease?

    a. Continue to work, but be careful.

    b. Have a physical examination to determine if a food handler is a carrier of a disease which could be transmitted to patrons or fellow workers; if so infected, a food handler may have to be furloughed or follow strict infection-control procedures.

    c. Wash hands frequently.

    d. Wear a clean uniform daily.

12. Name three serious diseases found in the workplace.

Salmonella, Hepatitis A, Ptomaine Poisoning, Botulism

13. All food service personnel are potentially exposed to which of the following?

Salmonella, Hepatitis A, Hepatitis B, Tuberculosis

14. In a clean kitchen area, which of the following describes why a need for effective disinfection exists.

    a. Microorganisms travel from areas which are not clean to those which are.

    b. Potentially infective organisms can exist on "clean" surfaces.

    c. Air-borne microorganisms settle on clean surfaces

    d. Microorganisms have no means of propulsion other than by people, objects, and air.

15. Which of the following governmental agencies is responsible for establishing and monitoring surface disinfectants and other cleaning and sanitizing supplies?

    a. EPA

    b. FDA

    c. CIA

    d. HEW

16. When glassware is improperly cleaned and stored, which of the following would most likely occur?

    a. Increased breakage

    b. Storage areas can become contaminated

    c. Beverage flavor would be affected

    d. Cross-infection of a customer can occur

17. Which best describes why the food service industry is constantly faced with Salmonella and other food-borne illnesses?

    a. It is impossible to prevent Salmonella in food handling and food preparation.

    b. Salmonella and Hepatitis A are transmitted by airborne microorganisms and air filters are not used to combat them.

    c. Appropriate and available infection-control measures are not used in the food service industry resulting in disease transmission.

    d. The problem does not actually exist, but is rather caused by over-reporting of a few isolated instances.

18. Food service areas can be either disinfected daily or routinely during the week depending upon the type of operation and the efficiency of the product used for disinfection.

True or False?

19. An infection-control program properly implemented would greatly reduce the risk of cross-contamination.

True or False?

20. When evaluating a disinfectant to be purchased, which of the following best describes the most important step?

    a. Check with current users of the product.

    b. Conduct cleaning tests to see if the product produces suds.

    c. Read advertising literature.

    d. Read the label on the container carefully to determine exactly which organisms the product kills or inactivates and that there is an EPA number certifying that the kill data are valid.

21. All chemical companies have been required by OSHA to provide which of the following to alert management?

    a. Cost of product at use-dilution

    b. Potential health hazards associated with use of the product (MSDS information)

    c. Time-temperature parameters for use

    d. Staining tendencies of various products

22. Personal hygiene is an important part of an infection-control program. Of the following, which best describes why there is concern about infectious diseases?

    a. We cannot eliminate human error nor can we monitor all steps in food preparation or handling.

    b. Inadvertently, improper hand washing may occur.

    c. Without the use of barrier protection like gloves, masks, aprons, etc., transmission can occur.

    d. Microorganisms do not discriminate; 20% of the population are carriers of some type of disease and the food service workers are not immune to infections which can be spread to others.

23. Which of the following best describes a high-risk area for disease transmission in a food service facility?

    a. Food handlers without immunization

    b. A food handler infected with Hepatitis A

    c. A food preparation area that has been improperly sanitized and exposed to blood from a nick while a food handler was slicing and overlooked the incident

    d. A freezer door handle touched by an employee after handling raw chicken

References

1. Gene Antonio, *The AIDS Cover Up*, Ignatius Press, San Francisco, California, 1986–1987, p. 113.

2. Steve Sternberg, from the Knight Ridder News Service, based on research by Dr. Resnick of Mount Sinai Medical Center, Miami, Florida, 1987 (*Journal of the American Medical Association*, volume 255, number 14, 1986).

3. Documented research available from the Centers for Disease Control, Atlanta, Georgia.

4. *A Clinician's Dictionary Guide to Bacteria and Fungi*, 4th Edition, revised, Eli Lilly and Company, Indianapolis, Indiana, 1981.

5. *Seattle Times*, April 13, 1987, Metro Edition.

6. *New York Times*, July 12, 1987, Sunday Edition.

7. *The Courier Journal*, Louisville, Kentucky, March 13, 1988.

8. Outbreak of scabies documented by a small community hospital, Pomerado Hospital, University of California Medical Center, San Diego, California.

9. W. Isaacson, "Hunting for Hidden Killers," *Time*, July 4, 1983, pp. 50–55.

10. 1987 Estimates from the Centers for Disease Control, Atlanta, Georgia.

11. *Morning News Tribune*, Tacoma, Washington, June 3, 1988; *Seattle Daily News*, "Fast Food Worker Exposed 5,200 to Hepatitis," Seattle, Washington, June 4, 1988, p. A1.

12. "Legionnaires: the Disease, the Bacterium, and Methodology," Centers for Disease Control Laboratory Manual, May 1978; revised October 1978, Atlanta, Georgia.

13. Centers for Disease Control, *op. cit.*

14. *Applied Foodservice Sanitation,* Third Edition, in cooperation with the Educational Foundation of the National Restaurant Association and the National Sanitation Foundation, John Wiley & Sons, Inc., New York, 1985.

15. George Schuler, G. Christian et al., *Food, Hands, and Bacteria,* University of Georgia, Augusta, Georgia, March 1980, Bulletin No. 693 (reprinted with permission).

16. *Federal Register,* Monday, August 24, 1987, Vol. 52, No. 163.

17. Ken Voit, Microbiologist, 1981 (unpublished); research in conjunction with CDC and University of South Carolina Medical Research Department; and *Morbidity and Mortality Weekly Report Summary of Notifyible Diseases, U.S., 1988,* published October 6, 1989 for 1988 Volume 37, Number 54.

18. N. B. Williams, "Microbial Ecology of the Oral Cavity," *Journal of Dental Research,* 42, 509–520 (1963), Supplement to No. 1.

19. *Morbidity and Mortality Weekly Report,* May 22, 1987, Vol. 36, No. 19, "Healthcare workers exposed to blood of infected patients," Center for Disease Control, Atlanta, Georgia.

20. Judy Grande, "What ails us is often in our food," *The Plain Dealer,* 1985 (reprinted with permission).

21. Educational Foundation, *Applied Foodservice Sanitation,* Third Edition, 1985.

Bibliography

Bond, Favero et al., "Inactivation of Hepatitis B Virus by Intermediate to High-Level Disinfectant Chemicals," *Journal of Clinical Microbiology*, September 1983, pp. 535–538.

Bond, Favero et. al., "Survival of Hepatitis B Virus after Drying and Storage for One Week," *The Lancet*, Volume 1, 1981, pp. 550–551.

Brandt, E., "Acquired Immune Deficiency Syndrome," Washington, D.C.: Memorandum from the Assistant Secretary for Health, Public Health Services, June 13, 1983.

Brown, Kathleen, and J.G. Turner, *AIDS: Policies and Programs for the Workplace*, New York, Van Nostrand Reinhold, 1989.

Centers for Disease Control, "Diagnosis and Management of Microbacterial Infection and Disease in Persons with Human T-lymphotropic Virus III/Lymphadenopathy-associated Virus Infection," *Morbidity and Mortality Weekly Report*, Volume 35, 1986, pp. 448–452.

Dykstra, J., *Everything You Wanted to Know about Infection Control: An Employee Training Guide on Infectious Diseases*, The J.D. Group, Inc., Infection Control Training Center, York, Pennsylvania, 1989.

Dykstra, J., "Proper Disinfection Is Your Business," *Food Service Forum*, Vol. 2, No. 3, December/January 1988.

Harris, J.E., "The AIDS Epidemic: Looking into the 1990's," *Technology Review*, Volume 90, 1987, pp. 59–65.

Institute of Medicine/National Academy of Sciences, *Confronting AIDS, Directions for Public Health, Health Care, and Research*, Washington D.C., National Academy Press, 1986, pp. 69–70.

Isaacson, Walter, "Hunting for Hidden Killers," *Time*, July 4, 1983.

Kilbrick, S., "Herpes Simplex Infection at Term," *Journal of the American Medical Association*, Volume 243, No. 2, 1980, pp. 157–160.

Olesbe, Minifer et al., "Immune Deficiency Syndrome in Children," *Journal of the American Medical Association*, Volume 249, No. 17, 1983, pp. 2345–2349.

Sistrom, William R., *Microbial Life*, New York, Holt, Rinehart, and Winston, 1969.

Susser, Peter, "AIDS: Legal Considerations," *The Cornell Quarterly*, Volume 28, No. 2, 1987, pp. 81–85.

Tanne, Janice Hopkins, "The Other Plague: Potentially Deadly Hepatitus B," *New York*, July 11, 1988, pp. 35-40.

Answers to Review Questions

Chapter 1

1. True
2. AIDS
   Legionnaires
   Cytomegalovirus
   Delta Hepatitus
3. b
4. d
5. c
6. True
7. To reduce the level of pathogenic microorganisms.

Chapter 2

1.	a	4.	a	7.	False
2.	a	5.	c	8.	True
3.	e	6.	False	9.	b

Chapter 3

1. c
2. Hepatitis, AIDS, Legionnaires'
3. c
4. a
5. b–best; a–also acceptable; c–a reality
6. All answers are correct; a is best
7. b
8. c
9. 2 to 1, Helper to Suppressor
10. Proteins, macrophages, and antibodies to fight off infection

Chapter 4

1.	a	4.	a
2.	b	5.	a
3.	b or d	6.	b

Chapter 5

1. Due to cross-contamination by cell slough from people. There is a need for some type of barrier protection due to constant exposure to germs in public places.
2. A liquid containing chemical energy capable of killing or inactivating certain microorganisms.
3. Must kill TB.
4. Labels state what claims are made based on required EPA tests. What is legally approved must appear on the label or container. Misrepresentation is illegal and appropriate ac-

tion (fines, cease and desist orders, imprisonment, and so on) results.

5. Cleaning assists in eliminating a large number of microorganisms and the organic matter may reduce the chemical energy of some disinfectants.

6. The chemical energy of the disinfectant is released while the product is allowed to air day (products like alcohol evaporate, quickly reducing its capability to eliminate many microorganisms).

7. Any form of the criteria will be appropriate. The most important is the TB kill factor, because this is the most difficult non-spore-like organism to eliminate without complete sterilization.

Chapter 6

1. True   5. False
2. False   6. d
3. False   7. a
4. c

Chapter 7

1. c   5. a
2. c   6. a
3. a   7. True
4. a or c   8. Rinse with potable water before reuse

Chapter 8

1. False   4. Yes
2. True   5. True
3. a. Former patrons
   b. Current patrons
   c. Future patrons

Chapter 9

1. True   5. True
2. True   6. d
3. c   7. d
4. Section VI

Review Self-test

1. b	10. d	17. c
2. a	11. b	18. True
3. c	12. Salmonella	19. True
4. c	Hepatitus A	20. d
5. d	Botulism	21. b
6. d	13. All	22. d
7. d	14. d	23. c
8. b	15. a	
9. b	16. d	

Index

A

Acquired Immune
    Deficiency Syndrome
    See AIDS
Aerobacter aerogenes, 20
Aging of America, 10
AIDS, 2, 5, 12, 39
    carriers, 43, 54
    contaminated needles,
        10
    infection, 39
    sexually transmitted, 10
    transmission, 12, 39, 95
    treatment, 40
    virus, 12
    virus carrier, 11
AOAC
    guidelines, 70
    standards, 70
Asepsis, 57–58
Aseptic
    definition, 18
Aspergillus species, 20
Association of Official
    Analytical Chemists
    See AOAC

Asymptomatic
    definition, 6
Autogenous infection, 18

B

Bacillus species, 20
Bacteria, 18, 21
    Actinomyces, 21
    Aeromonas, 21
    Bacillus, 22
    Borrelia, 22
    Diplococcus pneumoniae,
        22
    Enterococci, 22
    *Erysipelothrix
        rhusiopathiae*, 22
    Escherichia, 22
    gram-positive bacteria,
        119–120
    gram-negative bacteria,
        120
    Leptospira, 22
    Pseudomonas, 23
    Samonella, 23

Staphylococcus, 23
Streptoccus, 23
Treponema, 22
Bacteriostat, 93

C

Candida species, 20
Carrier, 18
Centers for Disease
    Control, 35–36, 39–40,
    45, 70, 75
    AIDS transmission, 95
    guidelines, 66
Clean, 93
Clean-room concept, 78
Cleaning procedures, 87
Communicable disease, 18
Container labeling, 141
Cross-contamination, 111
Cross-infection, 18, 112
    to travelers, 10
Cryptococcus species, 20
Cutaneous, 18

D

Dermatophytes, 20
Disease transmission,
    91–92, 117–118
    equation, 13
    mode of transmission,
    18
    prevention, 12
    route of transmission, 18
Disinfect, 3, 19, 59, 68, 73,

94, 107
    high-level, 4–5
    hospital-level, 4
    intermediate–moderate
        level, 4
    levels of disinfection, 4
    low–limited level, 4
Disinfectant, 65, 68, 124
    definition, 69
    high-level, 76
    hospital-grade, 65
    hospital-level, 71
    legal definition, 70
    product application,
        99–100, 124
    regulations, 67
    testing, 72
Disinfectant products, 96
    application, 96
Disinfection, 116
    high-level, 88
    procedures, 122, 124
    product application, 77
Disinfection solutions, 80
    advantages, 80–81
    disadvantages, 80–81

E

Employee Health Form,
    53–56
Employee training, 142
Endogenous infection, 18
Environmental Protection
    Agency (EPA), 3, 66,
    139
Escherichia coli, 20

F

Federal agencies:
  Association of Official
    Analytical
    Chemists, 70
  Centers for Disease
    Control, 70
  Environmental
    Protection Agency,
    69
  Food and Drug
    Administration,
    69
Fire Protection Checklist,
  152
Fomites, 18, 20
  definition 6
Food and Drug
  Administration (FDA),
  1, 14
Fungi, 24
  Aspergillus, 24
  Candida, 24
  Microsporum, 24
  Phialophora, 24
  Trichophyton, 24

G

Gram-negative bacteria, 21,
  65
Gram-positive bacteria, 21,
  65
Guest Room Checklist,
  132

H

Hand washing, 51
  technique, 52
Hazard Communication
  Program, 140–141
  company policy, 141
  container labeling, 141
  employee training and
    information, 142
  Material Safety Data
    Sheet, 142
Hepatitis, 35–36
Herpes I and II
  See Herpes Simplex
Herpes Simplex, 38
Hydrophilic viruses, 21
  Hepatitis, 21
  poliomyelitis, 21

I

Infection control
  checklist, 129
  fundamentals, 17
  guidelines, 115
  hand washing, 51
  high-risk employee, 56
  marketing, 15, 129
  marketing advantage, 14
  products, 79
  program, 14, 51
  protocol, 100, 125
  screening, 53
  seminars, 79
Infection-control program
  clothing, 51

goals, 7, 44–45, 90
hair care, 51

J

J.D. Group, 37, 79, 153
   Employee Health Form,
      53

L

Legionella
   See Legionnaires'
      disease
Legionnaires' disease, 36–37
Legionnellosis
   See Legionnaires'
      disease
Liabilities, 123
Lipophilic viruses, 21
   Herpes I and II, 21
   Influenza, 21

M

Marketing infection control,
   130
   certificate of
      attendance, 133
   direct mail, 130

infection-control
   checklist, 129
   to current patrons, 131
   to former patrons, 131
   to future patrons, 131
Material Safety Data Sheet,
   65, 142, 145–147
   checklist, 150, 151
   form, 147
Microbiology
   definition, 19
Microsporum species, 20
Modes of transmission, 25,
   27–29, 97
   cross-contamination,
      25–26
Mycobacterium species, 20

O

Occupational Safety and
   Health Act, 66
Occupational Safety and
   Health Agency
   See (OSHA)
OSHA, 11, 74
   authority, 97
   Employee
      Safety/Compliance
      Training, 154
   government
      intervention, 11
   Hazard
      Communication
      Standard, 65

inspections, 137, 139, 151
surveillance, 11

P

Pathogenic, 18
Pathogenic microbes
  Escherichia coli, 20
  Aerobacter Aerogenes,
    20
  Aspergillus species, 20
  Bacillus species, 20
  Candida species, 20
  Cryptococcus species, 20
  definition, 19
  Dermatophytes, 20
  fungi, 20
  gram-negative bacteria,
    20
  gram-positive bacteria,
    20
  Hydrophilic viruses, 21
  Lipophilic viruses, 21
  Microsporum species, 20
  modes of infection, 20
  Mycobacterium species,
    20
  Pseudomonas species, 20
  Salmonella typhosa, 20
  Staphylococcus aureus,
    20
  *Staphylococcus
    epidermidis*, 20
  Streptococcus pyogenes, 20
Pseudomonas species, 20

Q

Quaternary ammonia
  compounds, 81

R

Routes of transmission,
  25–26
  portals of disease entry,
    26–27

S

Salmonella, 43–44
Salmonella typhosa, 20
Sanitation, 116
  definition, 75
  related tasks, 105
  training, 106
Sanitize, 3, 19, 59, 69, 73, 93,
  107, 124
  industry definition, 19
  microbiological
    definition, 19
Sepsis, 18, 57–58
Serilize, 19
Staphylococcus, 20, 121
Staphylococcus aureus, 20
Sterilant
  definition, 69
Streptococcus, 20

T

Three-sink Theory, 113–114
    rinse tank, 113
    sanitize tank, 113
    wash tank, 113
Training
    checklist, 156–157
    J.D. Group, 154
    Test for Employees, 153

Training Checklist, 155
Tray cleaning, 109
Tuberculosis, 44

V

Virulence, 19
Virus, 18